From Bobcats to Rainbows

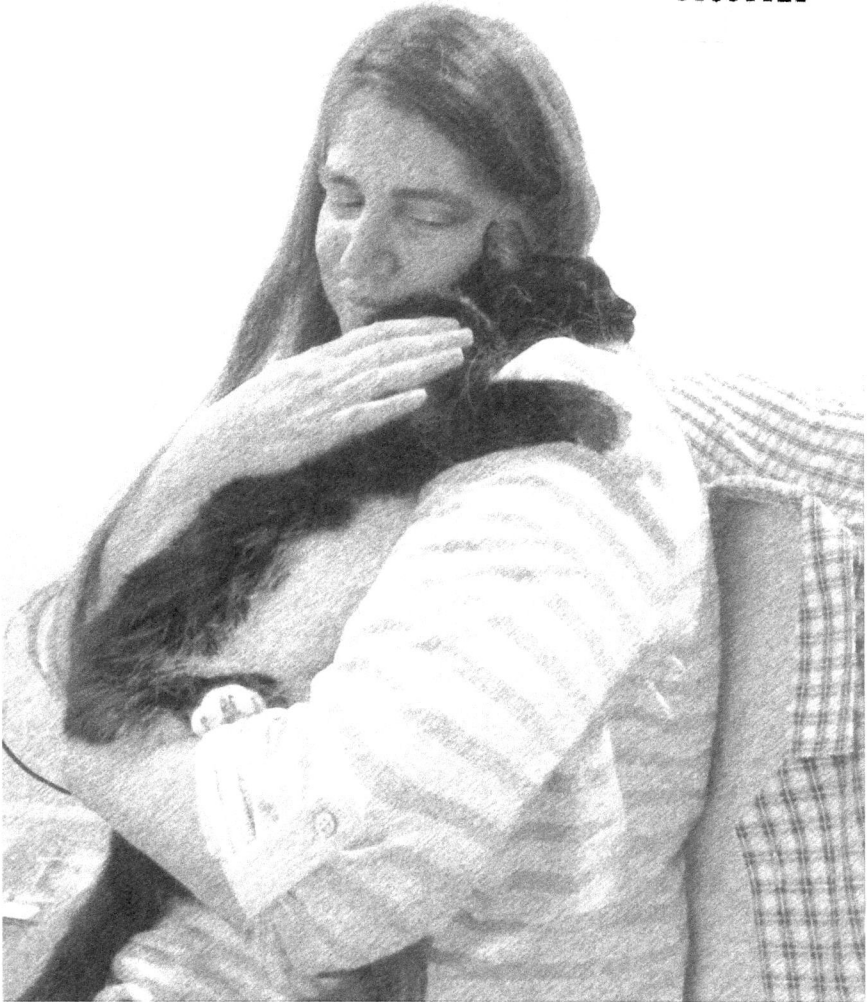

Michael Yanuck MD PhD

ISBN: 978-1-946600-46-2

DEDICATION

For Dr. Cami Zatkin,
the extraordinary veterinarian who cared for Cat Chow.

For Cat Chow's friend, Caroline Mccaffrey,
who loved Cat Chow and vice versa.

And for Cat Chow's mom and aunt,
April and Yael.

CONTENTS

FOREWORD

I'd been sharing this story as a "blog" and got the following response from my friend, Joyce.

"I just finished reading all your text about the end of life for cat chow," she wrote. "It sounds like she was a real happy healthy spirit, I don't think the spirit ever dies so I know she is somewhere waiting for you and April to rejoin her…"

Joyce had been the subject of many of my writings over the years. Perhaps a favorite for my readers was the story of her cat, Gizzy, an elderly cat that came with the house I'd rented from her. At that time, I'd had significant cat allergies, so I didn't think the arrangement was workable? However, Joyce assured me that I wouldn't have to physically interact with Gizzy, saying, "You don't have to worry, Mike. Gizzy is an outdoor cat. He never goes inside the house. All you have to do is give him some food. He won't bother you."

But then Gizzy became emaciated, as a result of arthritis and difficulty chewing, and I was concerned that he was starving? Again, Joyce reassured me.

"Sooner or later, Gizzy will simply wander off and find a solitary place to die," she said. "I've had cats all my life and that's what they all usually do."

But I didn't want Gizzy have to face mortality alone and, in spite of my cat allergies, took him into the house; and I just dealt with the allergic reactions, so that (long story short) on Gizzy's dying day, as I found myself reassuringly stroking his fur without experiencing any allergic reactions at all.

How had I overcome my cat allergies? Well, when I shared my Gizzy experience with a veterinarian friend, it was her opinion that the relationship with Gizzy had gradually tolerized me to cat dander, so that I'd developed an immunity.

"It's the same for people who get allergy shots," she said. "You get a little at a time until you develop a tolerance for the allergen. It sounds like that's what happened to you."

Joyce, however, was of a different opinion.

"Gizzy just figured you'd been so nice to him that he'd pay you back," she said.

And this takes me to my experience with Cat Chow: The experience with her had paid me back in spades! I'd learned to humble myself when relating to another; she provided companionship and comfort in one of my darkest hours; and in the end, she'd energetically imparted a dynamic internal Qi Gong practice that has the potential to reverse a lot of my persistent physical difficulties and benefit me for a lifetime.

I hope you'll find the sharing of this lived experience beneficial, too...

Disclaimer.

The author and publisher of this material are not responsible in any manner for any injury, physically or mentally, which may occur through reading or following the instructions in this book. The activities, physical or otherwise, described in this book may be too strenuous or dangerous for some people and readers should consult a doctor before engaging in them.

"Poor is the pupil who does not surpass his master."

— Leonardo da Vinci

1 INTRODUCTION

Urgent Phone Call...

On Friday, October 10, 2025, I got an urgent phone call from my main Native American collaborator, Chief Phillip Whiteman, who told me he has advanced stage cancer and wanted me to come to Montana and see him. He sounded weak, and I don't think he has long to live.

Phillip is a highly regarded and recognized Chief and Medicine Man who is frequently invited to speak in Native American conferences. During my years in South Dakota serving Native Americans of the Northern Plains, it was Phillip who literally sensed and intuited my training in Qi Gong, asking me what I knew about "energy"? When I told him about my Qi Gong training, he introduced me to Native American Medicine Men all over the Northern Plains, who shared many of their practices, which were not unlike Qi Gong; and Phillip urged me to share Qi Gong with them, as well, as apply it to help those in different native communities heal from the effects of historical trauma.

Most Energy Medicine agree that whether it's being practiced by Native American Medicine Men or Chinese Qi Gong Masters, they are all working at the level of the energetic circulation of the body.

The problem is, we know very little about Native American energy healing practices. To this point, previously I'd written three books, as well as numerous essays with Phillip, and, now, he wanted me to help him finish writing a final book about his practices that included energy healing.

This kind of opportunity was the reason I went to the Northern Plains in the first place and braved the harsh winters serving with native peoples as a physician and medical officer with the Indian Health Service. Hence, it was the opportunity of a lifetime, to say nothing of my desire to help Phillip, as matter of my regarding him as a close and dear friend.

"I love you, and send my love to your wife," he said, concluding the call. "And I'm thinking about you."

I loved you, too, I said, shaken...

CHAPTER ONE

Qi Gong and Native American healing interface...

I learned about a possible interface between Qi Gong and Native American healing practices while being considered for a position with the Indian Health Service. My recruiter was Dr. Dan Foster of the Rosebud Indian Reservation. When Dan learned about my Qi Gong training, he shared that he came from a long line of Lakota Medicine Men and had been involved in a study, which brought Lakota healers (like he and his brother) together with Qi Gong Masters from mainland China to compare techniques. According to Dan, by the end of the study, the Qi Gong Masters were deferring to the Lakota Medicine Men because they found the Lakota healing practices so much more advanced than their own.

After Dan told me this, I was hooked, and it didn't matter what anyone said or did thereafter; I was coming to the Rosebud Reservation.

Indeed, Dan wanted me to know all hard realities of the Reservation, and took my wife and me on a tour of the Rez that included trips to the sites of crimes like arson, robbery, and gang rape. As we drove, my wife looked on, horrified, and was surprised to find that no matter what Dan showed us, there was still a contented look on my face, as I just sat next to her, thinking, "I'm coming here. I'm coming here."

Nevertheless, when I began working at the Rosebud Indian Reservation Hospital, I expected it would take years of dedicated service before I'd established myself enough as a caring physician to be invited to the traditional healing ceremonies of the Lakota people I was serving. However, the tragic events involving a suicide cluster that occurred over the 2010 Memorial Day weekend would result in my being brought together with native healers much sooner than I could have ever imagined...

Over that Memorial Day weekend, I'd been out on the Reservation wading in the Little White River. I'd been enjoying being in the midst of the pristine nature of the Reservation, when suddenly I got caught in a veritable flash flood and had the good fortune of being pulled out of the river by some native men who saw me struggling.

Then, I went to the hospital and learned about the suicide cluster, presented in Morning Report as follows:

"Mary Eagle Heart. Eighteen years old. Found hanging by family members in their apartment. Died from cerebral edema brought on by hypoxia. It was later determined that the act occurred one year to the day after a sibling committed suicide the same way.

"Cynthia Black Horse. Nineteen. Overdose with respiratory depression and cardiac arrest. Coded. Unable to resuscitate.

"Wendy Sitting Bear. Eighteen. Suicide by slashing wrists.

"Donald Makes Room For Them. Found hanging. This following years of difficulties with alcohol and PTSD after returning from Operation Desert Storm.

"Rickie Kicking Bird. Eighteen. Shotgun injury to the head.

"Margaret Stone Calf. Eighteen. She was trying to commit suicide by getting run over on the road, and she was run over..."

These deaths left me stunned, especially as many of those who took their lives were young people who I had just watched graduate from high school. As a result, I felt it was imperative for me to assist at-risk youths and volunteered in suicide prevention programs.

At the same time, the tribe was inviting native healers from all over the Northern Plains to assist the children. Among those native healers was Phillip.

When he sensed my familiarity with Energy Medicine approaches, he shared that a knowledge of the energetic circulation has been known to native healers for centuries, and taught me that the horse possesses energy "sensors", which enable the horse to energetically connect with individuals and then help those individuals to correct their energy blockages for the sake of healing. In addition, Phillip showed me how to identify energy centers on the horse, and how their juxtaposition helped identify the personality, temperament and traits of the horse...

The Northern Cheyenne Reservation where Phillip lives has much the same conditions that led to the suicide cluster on the Rosebud Reservation: Unemployment, poverty, homelessness, suicide, alcohol and substance abuse, physical and sexual abuse, crime, arrests, incarceration, and, finally, poor medical care – the last of which I believe played a role in Phillip having wound up with advanced cancer.

At present, there was a problem, however; namely, Phillip wasn't the only significant relation in my life that was sick with cancer – and my cat (Cat Chow) also had cancer, and her lung cancer was getting worse.

Nevertheless, I immediately made plans to fly out to Montana and see him.

Calling him back about the flight, we made plans for my visit.

"When you come in on Saturday, we're going to sweat on Sunday," he said. "And then, the energy workers in Colorado with the Native American Church... That would be another opportunity to be exposed to that level of energy work."

I was surprised to hear that. I just thought the Native American church was about peyote. I didn't know they did energy work?

"Yes, it's more than that," he said. "We're going to drive down there to Colorado on the 23rd. You can ride down there with us..."

After the call, I spent the day with Cat Chow and my wife, April. April expressed concerns about Cat Chow.

"She's getting to a state where she's not able to purr easily," she said.

We'd been treating her with prednisone to keep her lungs open, but April expressed fear that the prednisone was just suppressing her cough, so that more secretions were collecting, and it was just going to be more "toxic."

I scanned Cat Chow energetically.

"I can feel the energy you're emitting to her," April said. "It's a calming energy.... No, really. Maybe that's why Cat Chow and Ini respond to you when they're really sick."

I thought about those times that I pulled Ini close when she was sick or injured, especially that night that she kept on having to go out to urinate every other second... That was the night I made the decision that I was taking Ini to the emergency room at UC Davis and she was diagnosed with that urologic malignancy that took her life not long after.

"Yeah, you're calming her down," April continued. "I think her breathing got better. She's not breathing as fast."

"What's the matter, Cat Chow?" I tried to say, lightheartedly. "You're not all feisty?"

"I think all the feist is out of her at the moment," April commented.

I made the mistake of stroking Cat Chow, and in response, her muscles tightened.

I told Cat Chow that I was sorry. I should have known better – and this right after talking with Phillip, who had trained me how to treat the "four-leggeds" with respect and humility.

"The horse is not impressed by status or fancy clothes or high-top sneakers," Phillip had taught, fifteen years ago. "He has no appreciation for those things. What he appreciates is the person inside. What he cares about is your intentions. He doesn't care about how much you know; what he wants to know is how much you care? And that's why you have to be respectful. That's why you have to be open. That's why you have to humble yourself to the horse. You have to want to serve, and not just one who is there to dominate, but one who comes to serve. And let those feeling guide you..."

CHAPTER TWO

Cat Chow...

Cat Chow had been having significant difficulties, as pertained to her lung cancer. Most of her difficulties revolved around episodic difficulties with being able to breathe, so that she'd at times she'd hunker down flat on the floor, gasping for air. In addition, there were extrapulmonary manifestations of the cancer, like a month ago (Friday, September 12, 2025) when I awoke at 2AM to the sound of Cat Chow scampering wildly all around the house. Cat Chow was an indoor-outdoor cat, so when she went to the bedroom's sliding glass door, I thought to let her out; however, there was something odd about the way she was walking – like she was having difficulty putting weight on her right leg.

"She probably finally jumped off of something and sprained her ankle," I thought.

But it was the first time that I'd ever seen Cat Chow have any form of physical difficulty. Our dog, Ini, suffered all kinds of physical injuries (a broken leg, torn ligaments, etc.), but, somehow, Cat Chow had gone through life without ever experiencing injury. So (for me), this was very unusual.

Getting up from the bed, I found that her behavior was odd, as well, because when I attempted to examine her, she rolled on her side, which was reminiscent of what Ini had done on those couple of occasions where she'd surrendered to fate, including when her leg was broken.

Frozen state, I thought. Possibly in the worst throes of pain.

So, I deduced there was something seriously wrong, and April and I put her in her kennel and drove to the Vet hospital.

Halfway to the hospital, I was rather questioning my decision, thinking, "Mike, what the hell are you doing? She probably just has a twisted ankle. Why are you treating this like an emergency? Are you out of your mind?"

Sadly, though, at the emergency room, the veterinarians diagnosed Cat Chow with something considerably worse than what I was expecting.

"Your cat has an arterial thrombus," the veterinarian told us.

An arterial thrombus is the worst kind of blood clot, because it cuts off the blood supply to distal tissues (in Cat Chow's case, her hind right limb).

"Given the high likelihood of gangrene and loss of limb, combined with her lung cancer, we recommend euthanasia," the veterinarian continued.

Now, when I was stricken with acute Covid about a year ago, I had an arterial thrombus, too – affecting my right hand, so that I was literally at risk of losing it. Cat Chow insisted on being with me back then; fortunately, my thrombus cleared, and, now, I wanted to fight for her to have the same outcome.

So, against the veterinarian's advice, we had Cat Chow admitted to the hospital for pain control (because of the horrible pain associated with the condition) and use of blood thinning agents to try to dissolve the clot. Fortunately, Cat Chow was lucky like me, and the clot cleared. However, coming back from the hospital, Cat Chow had problems of drop foot affecting that right hind limb; and she'd been so traumatized from the condition and the hospitalization, that she immediately went under the bed upon arriving home.

When she finally came out, April was quick to notice other changes.

"Her eyes are so open wide," she correctly, observed. "Especially around her irises."

Yes, her sympathetic nervous system was on overload, because of all the stress of the cancer and then the hospitalization.

Then, when she tried to jump off, and I went to stop her (fearing that she wasn't ready for that kind of physical activity, given the new problem of foot drop), she stopped in her tracks and laid down on her side, frozen again.

So, given her condition, I kept her by my side, as I performed external Qi Gong with her.

"She likes it when you do that with her," April commented.

Cat Chow lay on her side. It seemed she'd been having a very difficult time with the condition, which made sense, given how agile and mobile and independent and capable she'd been her whole life.

Except for the lung surgery five years ago to remove the cancer, she'd never been anywhere close to being physically disabled. Her whole life she'd really been able to enjoy her body, so this is a first for her.

Then, connecting energetically with Cat Chow, I experienced a stinging energy in my hand that ultimately went to the left side of my chest and it struck me that's where my heart is.

The energy then directed my hand back to her, with Qi emission occurring when my hand got close. In the process, Cat Chow was bit curious, but otherwise she accepting of it.

It was my great hope that Cat Chow would recover nerve function the way the Veteran (Kino) with left-sided neurologic deficits had in the Innovation Accelerator Qi Gong project.

And with time, Cat Chow mostly did recover function in that left back limb.

"Her paw was paralyzed, and they said that she wasn't going to get better," April said. "But then, it did get better, and she pretty quickly figured out how to use it. She is just so resilient. Whatever she wants to do, she'll figure out a way to do it. She is just so strong willed and strong.

"And she's willing to work with us. It felt like Ini wasn't as willing to that way and was more fragile somehow? She had a harder time healing than Cat Chow did. That's why in the end I was so reticent about doing that surgery on her. She just took longer to heal than anybody ever imagined, and there were always complications, and she was really suffering... She just had a really hard time with medical interventions and medical treatment. She almost always would have a bad side effect and this and that. While Cat Chow, she just likes sail through recovery. And she would recover in a way that the doctors couldn't even imagine that she could - Like five years after surgery for lung cancer, she's still alive, when they said that at most she would live for a year. She got back to full function after being told that she was going to lose her paw and it needed to be amputated - Like all of these different things that she would just sail through."

"She was just so strong," April concluded. "She knows what she wanted and she demands it!..."

CHAPTER THREE

Native American Energy Healing Session...

Phillip called back to tell me more about the energy healers who were going to be at the conference in Denver, and, in particular, the leading person for the Native American church, who had performed a previous energy healing on Phillip.

Phillip's significant other, Nicole, got on the phone and shared the details about the energy healing session.

"So, he also has it in his lineage from the Hidatsu people," she began. "He scans your body for anything that's wrong. For example, he found something behind chief Phillip's liver, where he was feeling his pain, where he had been punched and where everything kind of spread from. And chief Phillip hadn't told him any of this.

"So, he went behind him and sucked it out in a really traditional practice. And then he also used a kettle with coals in it, and crystals to look, and an eagle bone, and medicine to chew..."

CHAPTER FOUR

Spirit Buddies...

On Monday, October 13, 2025, Steve from our "Spirit Buddies" group called, and April shared that Cat Chow had a relatively good day.

"She keeps on going in and out, in and out today," she said.

"I think it's wonderful that she has this time with you," Steve said. "You're lucky. You're really, really lucky."

"I know," April agreed.

Then, she broke the news about Phillip.

"Mike's very, very good friend called us and said that he has metastasized cancer everywhere, so I urged Mike to go visit him, because I wished I had done that for Robert."

Robert had been April's boyfriend thirty years ago. He was Native American, and they had maintained a relationship all the way up to the time of his passing (though, sadly, he died unexpectedly, so she wasn't with him).

"So, Mike's going to go up to Montana for a week," she continued. "The sacrifice is, it's going to be time that he won't have with Cat Chow."

"That is true," Steve said. "But this is a friend, right? It's somebody who you've known for many years."

Yes, I'd known Phillip since my days at the Rosebud Reservation, when (after the 2010 Memorial Day suicide cluster there) the tribe brought Phillip to the Reservation to teach his native horsemanship practices to help at-risk youth.

And then Phillip took me under his wing and with him all over the Northern Plains, inviting me to learn Native American practices, and share what I knew about energy medicine practices.

April expressed her excitement, though she was wondering if it would be better if we waited until Cat Chow passed?

"But I think Mike is quite concerned that Phillip doesn't have that much time," she said. "And what's most important is that Mike does it before it's too late."

Steve asked when I'd last seen Phillip?

I said it had been over ten years: In December 2021 (after Ini passed), Phillip invited us to visit him and treat Ini's remains in the native American way. But then, my mother died just a couple of weeks later, and we didn't go.

In general, there was always an excuse for not going to visit him in the northern Plains: It's too far. It's too out of the way. And this time I felt like, "Enough excuses, I've got to do this now..."

CHAPTER FIVE

Delay of Care...

April lamented the advanced stage of Phillip's malignancy.

"But what I understand about cancer is, it doesn't show up until there are symptoms, and then when there are symptoms, it's too late," Steve commented. "And when you find that it's cancer, it's already everywhere. Isn't that just usually the case?"

"Well, Phillip was coughing and they didn't do a chest x-ray," April said.

Yes, he had described coughing for months and months, and just being treated with antibiotics and steroids, and a chest x-ray having never been performed.

Indeed, what prompted the chest x-ray that led to Phillip's diagnosis was his being physically assaulted while he was in Minnesota. It was for that reason (and not his other symptoms) that led to his undergoing the x-rays that turned up the masses in his lungs that would ultimately be found to represent widely advanced metastatic disease.

And then the origin of the cancer turning out to be from colon cancer, and his having never had or been offered a colonoscopy? That represented another flagrant source of malpractice. Because 15 years ago, Phillip had been diagnosed with psoriasis and been treated with immunosuppressive agents since then, and it was a known fact that medications like that predispose patients to cancer, because they partially turn off the immune system and, therefore, diminish the body's immune surveillance for cancer. Phillip was 67 years old. Regular screening colonoscopies begin at age 50. Hence, any medical professional with any sense would have recognized that and put it together and made sure Phillip had a screen colonoscopy he even got started on those drugs. It all just spoke of medical malpractice.

And now, Phillip said the doctors were bragging about him receiving the "best chemotherapy", but I'm just left to feel like, "Great, so they can bury you with a lot of the best chemotherapy."

"Yes, I understand the chemotherapy is great when the lesions are small and you can treat it, but not when it's advanced like that," steve correctly commented.

Yes, they weren't even taking out the source cancer in the colon. That's how advanced the cancer was.

"What's the point of even doing chemotherapy then?" Steve asked. "If it's already all over, and you can't even take out the cancer at the source, because it's metastasized and so advanced, would you go through all that radical chemo? Or would you just go on painkillers?"

According to Phillip, the chemo had stabilized his condition, so, at least, he lightheaded all the time from losing so much blood.

So, it wasn't like I disagreed with the treatment that Phillip was receiving; I was just grieving the delay of care. Because it was taking my friend out of this world sooner than could have been the case...

CHAPTER SIX

"Did not read the textbook..."

On Tuesday, October 14, 2025, I got news that the first article about the Long Covid-Qi Gong project was accepted for publication.

I felt a great sense of pride - With this paper, I would not only be recognized as an Energy Medicine scientist, but also an Energy Medicine practitioner of an approach that has helped those with a complex and complicated medical condition, for which conventional medicine is yet to come up with established and effective treatments.

Meanwhile, Cat Chow was having worsening problems: During the night, her breathing difficulties were worsening; and during the day, she wasn't eating or drinking as much.

Was the end getting close? I wondered.

At the time that I'd had these thoughts, I'd been watching her as she sat outside on the lawn chair that was draped by a lot of budding red flowers all around her.

Just then, she leapt down from the chair and came to the sliding glass door and rapped at the door. Letting her in, I was hopeful that she'd go to the kitchen to eat and drink; instead, though, she jumped on the bed.

Lying beside her, I heard gurgling sounds coming from her chest. I petted her, and she surprised me, because not only receptive to being petted, but when I stopped, she nudged me with her nose to continue, not unlike what Ini would do.

"Oh, how sweet," April commented. "She getting more cuddly with you."

Finally, I pulled my hand back in preparation to perform external Qi Gong, and energy filled my hand so quickly that I wasn't sure whether it was because I'd perceived an energy disturbance or I'd activated it with the energy myself?

In that moment, her breathing difficulties went silent, and whereas she's been purring before while I was petting her, now she was utterly quiet.

Then, to my surprise, I experienced an intense feeling of cold in my hand, so much so that it tingled and ached.

I recognized it as something I call the 'chill effect', which happens rarely in my energy work and usually goes along with attending individuals who are under considerable stress and strain.

The first time I encountered it was when I was working with Mrs. Ojeda (the mother of my "long lost love", Bubbles): At the time, Mrs. Ojeda was extremely ill, having suffered a heart attack and unable to eat because of an ulcer. Interestingly, near the end of performing BioEnerQi with her, my hands radiated with more energy than ever before, only to ultimately become utterly chilled!

"My hands are cold," I'd said at the time. "I mean, they're ice cold."

"Perhaps you've used up all your energy on me?" Mrs. Ojeda responded.

At the time, I stepped outside, and taking a short walk around the neighborhood in the afternoon sun, the frozen feeling dissipated.

Hence, now, with Cat Chow, I had no fear for myself when this occurred; I just wondered what this boded for Cat Chow?

The day before, April had commented that Cat Chow was different from Ini, in that Ini would pull back from energy work, whereas Cat Chow seemed to embrace it.

Then, as I lay next to Cat Chow, I noticed a feeling of tightness across my chest. I was hoping that it would result in spontaneous muscular releases and free up my chest more; however, the releases weren't coming; and what did come, was that thought that perhaps I should give Cat Chow some different food?

"Maybe she'll eat some of the canned wet food?" I thought.

Making my way to the kitchen, my mind drifted to thoughts of doubt.

"This is going to be futile endeavor," I thought. "She isn't eating because of the cancer. You went through all this just a year ago with Ini. The cancer is creating all kinds of acid-base and metabolic disturbances in her system. That's why she hasn't eaten or drank anything all day."

However, Cat Chow had followed me, and after I'd lovingly spread the contents of the can onto a plate, Cat Chow ate it all up and then drank some water.

"Perhaps it was the energy treatment?" I thought. "Maybe it helped her and that's why she ate and drank? And the feelings of physical discomfort and acting on them by getting out of bed and feeding Cat Chow was the right thing to do. And you should try not to question yourself so much, and get down on yourself when you don't get the kind of healing that you're expecting, and just because something doesn't happen as you would expect it would (like my expected muscular releases in response to the chest discomfort) doesn't mean that there's a problem - It's simply might mean that there's something else you need to do…"

Later in the day, April took Cat Chow for acupuncture (meant to help her with her leg).

"The vet said that Cat Chow was really amenable to treatment," April said on their return. "She said that Cat Chow was so chill during the acupuncture that she received today that she even permitted the acupuncturist to place a needle on her nose.

"And I said, 'Yes, she can recognize when something is good for her. She'll even jump on the bed and make it easier for me to get to her when it's time to give her her medicine.'

"And when we talked about Cat Chow's condition and her terrible prognosis and how she just keeps going anyway, the acupuncturist said, 'Cat Chow did not read the textbook'…"

I commented that Cat Chow was sleeping on the chair when I got home, and I was surprised that she didn't wake up when I went in and out.

"You know, she was like that this morning," April responded. "When I went to get her for her acupuncture today, she just let me pick her up. And before that I have been messing with her kennel, and usually that makes her run. But this time, she totally didn't pay any attention, and I walked right up to her and grabbed her, and she was like, 'Mom, what's going on?'

"But also, something really cute happened: When I got back, I let her out of the kennel in the car, and she jumped out, and then she walked with me all the way to the house door. Then, I opened the door and she went in.

"And it was very civilized. She walked with me, and I was like, 'Wow, it should have been on a video."

I nodded.

It seemed like Cat Chow's level of trust was just going through the roof.

"Yeah," April affirmed. "I was going to go to the store and get some more cat food, but I have the hardest time leaving the house because she was wanting me to pet her.

"I was at my computer, and she was behind my computer, wanting me to pet her head and neck."

Just then, Cat Chow went to April and did the same thing that she'd just described.

"And now she's doing it again!" April exclaimed.

April described a dream from this morning, in which she was with our dog, Ini.

"She was wagging her tail and her whole body," she began, "and I was really remembering all the details, so that it made me so sad that in my dream I got sad.

"So, I woke up, and then I noticed that Cat Chow had her tail on me. And I had this thought - because we know Cat Chow talks to the dead - So, I was wondering if I was getting Cat Chow's dream? It was like Ini reached out to me through Cat Chow?

"Because it was so real. I wish I hadn't gotten so sad, and I had stayed with it longer. But I got so sad. So, I woke up..."

CHAPTER SEVEN

Post-Study Qi Gong group...

On Wednesday, October 15, 2025, I began my Post-Study Qi Gong group by describing the call from Phillip and his telling me about his illness and asking me to come.

"Your friend wants to pass on this knowledge to you," ruth said. "And it's very important to him that he pass on that knowledge."

Ruth and the other members of this group were very wise. They'd been participants of the University of California-Davis Long COVID-Qi Gong study, in which I'd served as Qi Gong practitioner and succeeded beyond my wildest expectations in providing evidence that external Qi Gong imparted statistically significant improvements to long COVID sufferers for problems of fatigue, pain, activity intolerance, anxiety, depression and shortness of breath.

After the Long COVID-Qi Gong study, I'd suggested the Post-Study Qi Gong group, and Ruth and other study participants had been participating in it since.

Now, I confided to Ruth and the other members that I had reservations about going to Phillip: He had indicated that he didn't want to know his prognosis, and I was still grieving the passing of my dear friend and mentor, Sam, who had passed away just a few months earlier of a terminal lung condition and (in my opinion) didn't take advantage of learning enough about his prognosis to know what to expect, and I was afraid that would get in the way of honoring what Phillip wanted, because I was still mourning that when it came to Sam.

And there was more: I'd had a couple of dreams/visions involving Sam that I was having difficulty reconciling. Both involved my hairstylist, Jocelyn, who I regarded as an innate energy healer. I wound up sharing this opinion of Jocelyn with Sam years ago when Sam asked about my vision of heaven?

"Sam, I don't have a vision of heaven," I said. "It's not something that I particularly think about or reflect on."

"Oh, come on come on," he insisted, good-naturedly. "What's your vision of heaven?"

Oh, all right, I surrendered.

And looking to the side and opening my mind to my friend's request, instead of seeing pearly gates or a palace on a cloud, a vision of Jocelyn came into my head.

Ten years later, on the day he died, I awoke to a dream/vision of Sam OneWheeling into Jocelyn's salon. I thought, "What is he doing there? Well, maybe he went to talk with Jocelyn? I should probably give them some space." I turned and prepared to walk away, but then I thought, "I'd like to be in on the conversation and hear what they say." But turning around to go back, I awoke from the dream.

And describing that dream was the last thing I told Sam, as, afterwards, I went to work, as he'd requested ("Because you do important work," he said) and a few hours later, his wife texted that he had passed.

Then, the following morning, I had another dream/vision: This time of Jocelyn with a dark silhouette that possessed Sam's general physique, leading him away into the great beyond.

And that vision has been haunting me, because I didn't expect what amounted to Sam's spirit to be this dark silhouette. And I don't know what to do with that?

Then, I shared about an experience of connecting with Sam energetically over the Rosh Hashanah services while I was standing at the Torah and asking for a sign, and (long story short) I had the feeling that the hereafter was a place of darkness that didn't seem like all that much fun, so to leave me less than confident about wanting to go to there, and feeling like (when that eventually happened) I'd like to return to the physical plane again, and, thus, maybe the physical plane and the spiritual plane were intertwined and connected, and the spiritual plane is invested in the physical plane? And that, in turn, left me feeling like I had to re-double my efforts to make the world a better place.

"Your dream is very real," Ruth commented. "And very meaningful. But just remember that don't let your dream interfere. I mean, it's very hard, and it's very real. But don't let your dream interfere.

"My mother said when she was very sick, she wanted to know that I would do well after she left. And moments of grief were acceptable, but not to let it interfere with our time together."

"I am just so honored for you," she continued. "That he wants to give you this wonderful gift. This can change your whole life – This may change your whole life - Again…"

I shared about Phillip how it was that he had the greatest heart. He was fearlessly giving, just like Sam was. He didn't let fear get in the way.

And so many of my friends that way. They were almost otherworldly in their ability to give of themselves. They would put themselves in compromise positions in order to give.

Whereas I felt I would not, and if I felt there was a danger in being giving, I would pull back, and wouldn't chance being struck in order to help someone, thus, making me more careful.

"And that's something that we love about you," Ruth responded. "So, don't fault yourself for that…"

CHAPTER EIGHT

Phillip and Sam intertwined?

Interestingly, the Qi Gong session that began with me talking about Phillip posed against my recent experience with Sam, mostly ended with my "connecting" with Sam, as leading the Qi Gong self-practice entering a Qi Gong state, in my eyes, the darkness that I'd seen in Sam's silhouette became crystal clear and beautiful, so that I could imagine enjoying my time there.

My hands were full of energy and reaching to the sky as I had this vision; and as I stood with my eyes closed emersed in this energy, I described Sam's Celebration of Life, and the comic cartoon images of Sam that had been planted in several vases full of flower; and how Sam's daughter had permitted me to take a couple of them home, and the ones I chose were with him with his Rubiks cube, and then another with him training a chimpanzee to ski.

I described Sam's irreverent humor, and how it was that when the pastor had asked Sam how he wanted his Celebration of Life to be conducted, Sam had suggested putting his ashes in a piñata and then letting everyone attending take a swing!

He was cool, calm and collected and full of fun.

"He said, 'Everything in moderation'," his daughter recounted at the Celebration. "'Except fun,' he said. That was the exception…"

My wonderful, wonderful, wonderful spirit of a friend, I said. I couldn't wait for him to not be in pain anymore in this life, but how I wish you were here to help me understand that last vision.

He didn't believe in God or religion, but told me not to worry about him, and, "It was just a walk in the forest. It was just another path."

Listening, I'd hope he was reassuring to himself, because his mortal self was deteriorating before our eyes, and he knew that he now had to leave the physical plane – That was for sure, and it was time. It was definitely time.

And with that thought, the energy left my hands (though it was still in my head, especially my third eye, upper third eye, and crown chakra).

My eyes still closed, I stopped sharing about my thoughts and experiences and inquired about how Ruth was doing? And found that she wasn't there and, for the first time in a year of doing these virtual Qi Gong sessions, the internet had got disconnected...

CHAPTER NINE

Intent on coming to Montana?...

As I packed my things for the trip to Montana, Cat Chow jumped on the bed and got into my half-packed suitcase, as though saying she was intent on going with me to visit Phillip.

Already, Cat Chow had been in the habit of jumping into the bed and looking back and inviting me to join her.

A year ago, when I'd been seriously ill with acute Covid, Cat Chow had been insistent on being with me. At the time, April didn't want Cat Chow to be in contact with me (because cats can contract COVID-19). But Cat Chow would not stop scratching at my door, and, ultimately, we let her in, so that she could be with me.

And when I was experiencing fever and chills and that arterial thrombus in my arm, she was right there with me.

And, now, I wanted to be there for her...

Turning to April, I shared these feelings and said it only seemed right that I was now there for her in whatever time she had left.

"But you are, in a sense," April replied. "You're not making her move."

Yes, where the veterinarians had informed us that Cat Chow was not in any state to make the trip to Connecticut (where I had plans to start a research fellowship in external Qi Gong), we'd made the decision that April and Cat Chow were going to stay here in California for the duration of her life.

"And who knows how long it's going to be?" April added.

April turned to Cat Chow.

"You're not making a move," she told her. "You don't have to get used to a new place."

April added that she'd talked with the physical therapist, and that person affirmed the veterinarians concern about moving Cat Chow in anyway.

"Even the drive is very stressful for cats," she said. "You know it was very stressful for her coming out here."

I thought about how it was that Cat Chow's meowing was the source of company during the trip, and now all I could think about was what a terrible torture it was for her and how insensitive I'd been and just imagined myself in the throes of those panic attacks that I experienced with acute Covid, and then being locked in a cage for hours and days the way Cat Chow was.

"You remember about halfway through, that's when both Cat Chow and Ini just gave up any pretense of being strong," April recalled. "It was on the Green River, right?"

Yes, in Wyoming (which, as fate would have it, would be the State where I'd find myself on this trip, when Phillip unexpectedly took me with him to a place called Thermopolis!).

"They were like, 'You're not going anywhere without us'," April continued.

Yes, Ini would bark through the door if we left together to get breakfast in the main lobby of the hotel without her.

"That's when we had to split up to go for breakfast," she said. "One of us had to stay with them at all times - Because they were just done!"

With Cat Chow, it was actually well before that – in Ogallala, Nebraska. There, while April was busy doing the laundry, I opened the door to our motel room, and Cat Chow stealthily sprang from the couch and made like a bullet through the door to the outside.

"No, Cat Chow," I cried. "You don't want to do this. You are miles from home. Please come back."

My arms outstretch and extended and lurching after her like some Frankenstein's monster, I followed Cat Chow around the parking lot, pleading with her to return to the room.

But it was to no avail, as Cat Chow just increased her distance from me, till finally I gave up and went to April and confessed what happened.

"She's angry at us," April said, understandingly. "That's why she did it."

Yes. For the past days I'd kept her in that cat carrier, in spite of her objections. Now, this was the result.

"The only way that we're going to catch her," April continued, "is if she wants us to. Believe me, I know this from experience. She's a very fast and very capable cat. I've known this for a long time about her. I can't catch her. I am not fast enough or have good enough reflexes to catch her. If I catch her, it either means that she wants or is letting me catch her.

"It's going to be up to Cat Chow whether she comes back to us, or not. She has the choice right now. It's her choice. Either she chooses to come back to us, or she chooses not to. It's her choice. We lost control of the situation. She has control of it now. We're just going to have to let her stay out for a while, Mike."

Still beside myself and feeling like an utter failure, I shook my head disparagingly and returned to the room.

It was all my fault, I thought, and now Cat Chow was likely lost to us forever.

April stayed outside, though, gently calling to Cat Chow.

"Cat Chow," she called. "Cat Chow..."

Then, about an hour later, Cat Chow came through the open the door into the motel room, with April following her.

"You know why she followed me?" April said. "It's because of the past year. Over the past year I've developed more of a relationship with her. If this had happened the year before while we were coming from Chamberlain to Rockville, I don't think she would have come back. But after this last year, there is enough of a bond of trust between us that she was willing to come and follow me back."

"I guess I'm becoming a real cat whisperer," April declared...

Yes, our lovely, four-legged companions – They were with us by choice, and were the treasure of our lives...

CHAPTER TEN

Yellow Horse...

Saturday, October 18, 2025

Arriving at the airport in Billings, Phillip was quick to pick me up, and we were immediately off to purchase supplies in town, which found me hauling 50-pound sacks of grain into his trailer.

Next, we went to a lumber yard, where some 500 pounds of tree parts were loaded by a forklift into the bed of Phillip's truck – This to be used in the wood stove that heated his home, as well as to fire the stones used for the next day's sweat lodge ceremony.

A night's rest was followed by full day of backbreaking work of chopping the 500 pounds of wood and tending all of Phillip's herds of horses, cattle and buffalo. As I worked along Phillip, we were thankfully joined by members of Phillip's family, as well as young people from the high school. In that regard, I particularly appreciated this student, Michael, for his humility, and a young family member, Chance, for his strength and charisma.

The Sweat Lodge ceremony happened after sunset: Those present talked about their lives, which were full of problems and hardships, grief and struggles, most of them seemingly self-inflicted by embracing simple pleasures that went off the rails, like too much drinking and sex, leading to physical and sexual abuse, crime, arrests, incarceration, children and custody fights!

Even Phillip attested to these difficulties himself, admitting that (between at least three women) he had ten children, and it didn't sound like any of them were in any place to carry on his teachings and legacy?

As the ceremony progressed, with water poured over the hot stones and prayers offered, I considered the state of affairs on the Reservation: On the Northern Cheyenne Reservation (like most Reservations), the unemployment is 80-90% (as was the rate of alcohol and substance abuse), resulting in poverty, homelessness, and suicide.

Then, there's the poor medical care, which I believe played a significant role in Phillip having wound up with advanced cancer.

Then, just before the end of the ceremony, Phillip announced that he was giving me a Cheyenne name: Heovo'hame (Yellow Horse), which had belonged to one of his eight great grandfathers who fought in the Battle of the Little Bighorn (not far from his home).

I asked if the name had any meaning or significance beyond having belonged to his great grandfather?

"Yes," Phillip responded, emphatically. "When the golden sun rises in the morning, it brings life; and when the golden sun sets in the West, that's the future looking back at us. A yellow horse is the one that's going to carry you through that journey..."

CHAPTER ELEVEN

External Qi Gong & Qi emission...

After the Sweat Lodge ceremony, I asked I could attempt to help Phillip by performing external Qi Gong?

Phillip insisted I do this first with his significant other, Nicole, because he wanted to see how I did it with Nicole before working with him.

Connecting with Nicole energetically, I experienced a feeling of energy on the right side of her chest. And the energy kept me there. It didn't move.

Nicole described how it was that the energy interaction was eliciting a feeling along the right side of her mid back, where she typically feels tension when someone is "stabbing me in the back" as pertains to her previous life in Europe.

Interestingly, I was also feeling energy at my left hand interacting with my solar plexus.

Finally, the energy at my right hand, let go, and at that moment, I experienced the activation of my crown chakra.

And when the energy at my left hand let go, I still felt energy the activation of my solar plexus.

Nicole said she felt lighter, and, in addition, to feeling the release of tension along her right back, and she said that a headache she'd been experiencing went away.

Next, I worked with Phillip. The energy interaction was interesting: It began with my perceiving energy at Phillips chest. But it was much more than this, because it felt like there was energy moving from my hand into Phillip's chest! And this "sending energy" was very different for me, because there was nothing about seemingly integrating the energy that was coming from him, and then sending it back (which was my usual and accepted pattern if I performed Qi emission). It was just right away – BOOM – I was sending energy to him.

Again, this was like nothing I'd ever done before. The energy was just flowing to him, and it reminded me of that dream that April reminded me of before I left for the trip… Of the Native American man with whom I fused into the doorway.

Looking out at the rugged beauty of the Great Plains I heard the sound of Lakota drums and chanting. A large Native American man stood in a doorway; framed against a clear blue sky, he appeared weak and dehydrated.

"Water. Water."

Running to him, I heard my fiancée call to me sweetly. For a moment I turned to look back, then redirected my gaze, and hastened my step.

But the suffering man had transformed, his very substance having fused with the door, so to appear like some carved figure in the wood. And reaching him, I, too, transformed — merging and coalescing with him into the doorway…

Finally, it felt like I stopped sending energy to Phillip, and, instead, I felt energy at the back of my fingers.

When I describe this, Phillip said that he was now feeling energy on the palmer surfaces of his fingers, which had become discolored because of the chemotherapy, just like the souls of his feet.

Following the energy path, it directed me backwards, and I experienced a feeling of tension at my right inguinal area.

I wondered if it had anything to do with Phillip, like he was suffering from a inguinal hernia, or had a previous inguinal repair because of our rodeo accident?

Phillip responded this was not the case, though he'd had appendicitis and an appendectomy.

That didn't feel like it quite represented what I was feeling.

Then, I felt this significant ache all over the upper part of my right leg, like something was really working itself out, perhaps mostly in the area of the adductor muscles?

Then, I felt this great sense of release of tension in my solar plexus that just felt really good, almost to the point of euphoria.

It was just such a terrific feeling of freedom and joy, and as though he were saying to me, "Don't worry so much about things and just do what you think is right."

Phillip said that he felt very light afterwards and like I was there to help him with his cancer and chemotherapy...

CHAPTER TWELVE

Glad I went?...

"So, are you glad you went?" April asked.

Of course I was. I was enjoying all of Phillip's animals, from his lovely doggies who are so friendly and soulful, to his horses, and cattle, and buffalo.

I was also seeing firsthand that Phillip was (in my opinion) working too hard for a 68-year-old man with advanced malignancy.

I'd looked up the prognosis of metastatic colon cancer and found the five-year prognosis was 10%.

Nevertheless, being on the Reservation again was to me like being in the Garden of Eden.

And I loved being with the kids here, who I found pleasant and respectful and a joy to be with.

"I told you you should have gone and visited him," she said. "You should spend time with him every year..."

CHAPTER THIRTEEN

Feeling rather than thinking...

The following day, I raised the issue with Phillip that I don't really have any concept what I'm doing when I perform energy healing beyond connecting with the energetic circulation and following where it leads.

"So, I have no idea what's really happening," I said.

Phillip responded that when he would ride horses, rather than think, he would feel.

"So, whenever I stopped feeling what was going on, and started thinking, that's when I would get bucked off," he said. "And I wasn't bucked off a lot. Maybe a handful of times. I can count on my hands how many times I was bucked off.

"Fear and adrenaline are twins. One of them is telling you, 'You're not ready', and the other one is telling you, 'You're more than ready.'

"So, when you start thinking in fear, that means you're not ready. You're not prepared.

"But when you just let go and feel, and you feel that adrenaline, you're ready. You're more than ready. If you've done the preparation, and you've done the work you're supposed to do to get yourself in shape and have done all the necessities, you're ready.

"And you cannot lie to your body, because it's a body of truth.

"Your body knows, if you didn't put your time in, you didn't put your work in, then you're not ready to get on, and that's when fear disguises itself sometimes as adrenaline.

"And adrenaline sometimes disguises itself as fear," he concluded.

Then, he shared an experience of self-sabotage.

"When I went to Pendleton Round-Up... Well, not just anybody gets to ride at Pendleton Round-Up; you got to earn a certain amount of money in order for them to accept your entry. And then just because they accept your entry, you're not guaranteed to ride there.

"So, when I had won a certain amount of money, so I decided to go ride at Pendleton.

"And that Pendleton Round-Up really showcases its Indian people, because of that 'Happy Canyon' [side show that depicts the American West, beginning with a portrayal of early Native American culture, to the arrival of Lewis and Clark]. When I was a child, my parents took me there, and I went there as a participant at Happy Canyon and the parade and the powwow. I even won first place in my category and received an honor, so that my father got a horse.

"So, to go back years later as a true professional saddleback rider... Well, that's like unheard of. For an Indian to be a bona fide professional Bronc rider and be riding at Pendleton - The highest honor in a Pro Rodeo.

"So, I entered it, and my entry was accepted. And I was so excited. I put the two and two together: If I ride, and even if I buck off, I already won. I already won. To actually participate at Pendleton, and then being an Indian, and then being a winner in the other arena - the powwow arena - and now I'm riding in this arena. I'm already a champion.

"So, I'm thinking that way. And when I went to the entry office, the rodeo secretary was sitting there, and I waited in line, and there was a young man who fell off a horse the day before, and he had a broken leg, but and the blood clot went to his heart, and he died this morning. So, they were passing around a card and asked everybody to sign it. So, I signed it, and I signed it, 'World's champion Indian bronc rider, Phillip Whiteman.'

"And then the lady looked at me and noticed I was an Indian, and said, 'The Indians enter over there. That's where the Indians enter for the wild horse race.' And I said, 'I know that, but I'm not in the wild horse race, and I'm not in the powwow; I'm in the rodeo. I entered through PROCOM, out of Colorado. And I have my protocol entry form number if you want to see that.'

"So, she said, 'What is your name?' So, I said, 'My name is Phillip Whiteman.' And she looked and looked through the list and said, 'I don't see your entry. I don't see your name on the entry list.' And I looked at her and I said, 'Can you please look again? Because, by all rights, I should be the only Whiteman entered at this rodeo today.'

"And then she looked at me and she just stopped, and she said, 'Oh, there you are. I see you.' So, she gave me my badge number, but then she delayed me. She delayed me! And by the time I got to the back of the Bucking shoots, the security guard said, 'No Indians allowed behind the bucking shoot', and pointed to the other side where the powwow was happening. 'That's where the Indians sit, over there.'

"And I said, 'No, I'm here as a contestant.' I showed him my badge number. And they said, 'Oh, well, you could have just picked that up from the ground.'

"Then, he says, 'And the saddle that you're carrying – What's that for?' And I said, 'I'm a contestant. I'm probably supposed to start any minute.'

"And pretty soon I heard somebody saying, 'Phillip, get in here. Your horse is waiting for you.' So, finally, they let me in there. But the security guard followed me. And some of the other contestants were asking me, 'What are you here for? You should go back to Indian rodeos. You don't belong here.' And I was getting on my horse, and they were all standing back there, looking at me.

"And then finally, I rode my horse, and my horse came out really bucking, so that when it touched that grass, it took off running. And I was riding that horse across that arena that was running full blast. So, when it touched the ground on the other side of the track, it started bucking again.

"And hear the people start stomping their feet, so that it just shook that whole arena, because when a contestant deserves a re-ride, that's what they do: they stomped their feet.

"So, I got a re-ride. But by that time, I was already so angry that when I got back to the shoots and had my horse all ready, then once I tapped off on it, after the second or third jump, I just started over exposing myself. I wasn't even in the saddle: I was just mainly using my feet and my reins to stay on. And I was doing it to show them that I belonged there. I belonged at that level. And then the next thing I knew, just right before the whistle blue, the horse stood me up in my saddle, and I was standing alongside of it. It didn't buck me off; I spurred myself off. Because I wanted to overcompensate for the racism and the oppression and the discrimination that I felt, not only from the secretary, but from the security, and from those contestants..."

CHAPTER FOURTEEN

Origins of Whiteman name...

Phillip shared the origins of his last name.

"My great-great-grandmother, Vonha, was raped by a US soldier," he began. "She was thirteen when it happened. That was common - They went after girls that age to avoid venereal disease.

"So, when my great-grandfather was born, they named him, Vehoc, which means spider or trickster, because it was the way the Cheyenne referred to white people. Christian missionaries translated it to 'Whiteman', since his father was a white soldier.

"My great-great-grandmother could have abandoned him. People told her, 'He's theirs. Let them raise him.' But she loved her son and raised him Cheyenne. It taught me you can either hate and abandon, or you can accept and love, and my great-grandmother chose the latter path.

"By the time of the Sand Creek massacre, Vonha had already had another baby by a Cheyenne man, so, again, they said about Vehoc, 'Leave him. He's one of theirs. They'll take care of him.' So she was waiting to hand her baby to a man who was on horseback; but, instead, he grabbed the baby by the side of his face, and ripped it, so that he had a scar for the rest of his life.

"After she perished because of everything going on in the Black Hills, her sister took over as Vehoc's mother. She was later massacred with hundreds of others at Wounded Knee and still lies buried in the mass grave.

"When Vehoc was a young man, he fought at the Battle of the Little Bighorn. My father's grandmother, Quill Dress Woman, was a little girl at that battlefield and witnessed Cheyenne mothers push sewing awls into Custer's ears – So that the next lifetime he would listen. They did this because after the Washita massacre, where Custer attacked and killed defenseless women and children, our Cheyenne chiefs still made peace with him. In the sacred pipe ceremony, the chiefs told Custer to rub the ashes from the pipe into the ground, and warned him if he ever double-crossed the Cheyenne again, he would end up like those ashes. Custer didn't listen, but what the chiefs told him came true.

"After their defeat at Little Bighorn, the 7th Calvary and the Army made extermination our people their top priority. They said all our people had to be resettled in the south, in Oklahoma, even though, by treaty, our homelands were in the north. They said it was for our own protection and promised us, if we didn't like it in Oklahoma, we could go back.

"And, sure enough, in Oklahoma, our people wound it sick and facing starvation. So, our chiefs, Dull Knife and Little Wolf, told the white administrators they were going to take the people back to our homelands in the north. But, now, the white administrators said they couldn't do that, and couldn't go back, and they just had to stay put.

"So, Dull Knife and Little Wolf took the people north, anyway, because if they didn't, there wouldn't be any of us left. And the US army came after them and hunted them down like dogs.

"When the Army caught up with Dull Knife, he imprisoned his group in jail cells at Fort Robinson. For days, they kept them locked up without food or water or heat, and told them they'd stay like that, until they promised to 'voluntarily' return south.

"But rather than return south to more sickness and starvation, our ancestors broke out of their cages and made a run for it. Many of them were slaughtered right there on the spot – Shot point blank wherever the soldiers found them.

"The few who survived kept moving northward, for hundreds of miles, wounded, until they finally got reunited with Little Wolf and our ancestors on my father's side, and made it home north.

"And because of everything they went through, and that was done to them, and all the bad press it got in the newspapers at the time, the government established the Northern Cheyenne Reservation, for the survival of our way of life.

"That's why for the last 30 years I've led the Fort Robinson Breakout Run: So, our Cheyenne children could know what their ancestors went through, and run 400 miles in their footsteps, through four states and in the harsh winter conditions.

"And it's amazing to see them work together and find themselves. Alcohol, drugs, suicide are merely symptoms of oppression. When they run, they remind themselves of the spirit, resilience and sacredness of our Cheyenne ways..."

CHAPTER FIFTEEN

Encounter at Rosebud...

During the night, we traveled to Wyoming, where Phillip had a meeting planned with Arapahoe and Shoshone tribal representatives and community partners to resolve an ongoing dispute involving a sacred hot spring in Thermopolis.

"The hot spring there had been a place where all the tribes could meet in peace and get healing there," he said.

As we made our way along the highway, we passed the site of the Battle of the Rosebud, Phillip pointed out that ancestors from his family had fought here, as well.

"This is where the young girl saved her brother," he commented.

Indeed, I was to learn that the Battled of Rosebud was referred to as the Battle Where the Girl Saved Her Brother by the Cheyenne because of an incident during the fight involving Buffalo Calf Road Woman.

"It's because when Buffalo Calf Road Woman heard her brother, Chief Comes in Sight, had been wounded and left for dead, she went riding out into the battlefield at full speed and grabbed her brother and carried him to safety," Phillip said. "They say that the first and only time the US Army was defeated was the Battle of the Little Bighorn. But it was actually here, at the Battle of Rosebud that it happened first," he continued. "Just right here. Imagine the victory. Imagine the whooping and hollering. It was just the Cheyenne. No Lakota. No Arapahoe. Only Cheyenne."

We stopped and got out of the truck to pay our respects.

After keeping my head bent for a while in silent prayer, I looked for Phillip. Nicole told me he was relieving himself. I considered joining him, but also considered where I was standing, and wondered if it wasn't disrespectful? Then, I decided I didn't know how long we would be traveling and better do the same.

I separated myself from Nicole, and, feeling alone in the darkness, undid my fly.

Then, I heard something.

"Animal!" I yelled and ran in the direction of the truck. "Animal!"

As I ran to the truck, Phillip went running towards me. Ultimately, shining a light into the darkness, we found a lumbering, big, white cow.

Phillip doubled over, laughing.

"The way you were screaming, my first thought was a grizzly bear got you," he said, still laughing. "My second thought was a mountain lion got to you. But it turns out that it was just a jersey cow that heard you and probably came towards you because it needed to be milked..."

CHAPTER SIXTEEN

PTSD for the enemy...

Considering our conversations about his ancestors in battles like the Little Bighorn and my cowardice on the road, I was reminded of thoughts I'd had 15 years ago while visiting the Little Bighorn Battlefield National Monument for the first time. I was with April then, and reading the placards describing the different skirmishes between the Seventh Calvary and Lakota and Cheyenne and Arapaho on that fateful day, June 25th, 1876, I got out of the car and dropped to my knees and told April, "I can't imagine the fighting that occurred here… Men killing each other. The fear they must have experienced."

"And then, she said, 'I could imagine Phillip fighting here'," I said, continuing the story. "And I thought, 'Of course. Fearlessly taking to a horse – in a hail of bullets – charging into battle to protect his people. He would do this. He would have done it a hundred years ago. He battles for his people now.'"

To my surprise, rather than accept April's compliment, Phillip acknowledged my feelings.

"Until the day he died," Phillip responded, "my great grandfather had trauma – PTSD – because he saw those young soldiers killing themselves – shooting themselves and taking poison that day.

"We Cheyenne are a peace-loving people. We would have taken those young men, instead of killed them. And, so, my great grandfather kept waking up from his sleep, haunted, by the young white men who killed themselves rather than surrender.

"He was a very powerful Medicine Man at the time of the battle. He wasn't young. My mother was born in 1926, and she was about 10 or 11 years old when he died. So, go from 1876 to about 1936, and that's like 60 years after the battle, and in all that time, he was still waking up to that."

Nicole was not as magnanimous.

"But when I pick sage on the battlefield," she said, "I think, 'Fertilized by Custer'..."

CHAPTER SEVENTEEN

A calming influence...
Monday, October 20, 2025

For a short time, on the way to Wyoming, there was enough to reception to be able to take another Spirit Buddies call with Steve and April.

April talked about Cat Chow and what she'd done before I left for the trip.

"She was being so sweet," April told our friend, Steve. "She spent all night inside of Mike's open suitcase."

Yes, I'd left the suitcase on the right side of the bed, and slept on the left side, so that Cat Chow could remain in the suitcase.

"Maybe she wanted to leave her scent on Mike stuff?" she said.

Updating Cat Chow's condition, April commented about how it was that, in many ways, Cat Chow responded better to me than to her.

"Because I'm something of a Nurse Rached with Cat Chow," she said. "I nurse medicine down her throat. And I'm a lot less respectful of her, because I sometimes have to grab her and put her in the kennel. I'm the one who takes her to the doctors. So, I'm a little bit more physical with her.

"And Mike is more respectful of her 'cat distance', so they will do things like hang together, but he won't force her to let him pet her or do anything like that. He'll just let her hang around next to him, which she really appreciates.

"Early on in the relationship, because of the way that she would get angry at him and punish him, he became very respectful of her wishes. So, if she wants to go out, he immediately lets her out. Like

41

he's very responsive. And I'm not. Sometimes I'm like, 'I don't want to, Cat Chow. You'll just have to deal with it.' But Mike will immediately open the door for her.

"And most of the time, on a day-to-day basis, I think my approach is very practical, because I run the clinic, and sometimes she doesn't wanna do things, but she needs to do them, and I do those things.

"But at a moment of crisis, like emotional crisis, like she was in when she came back from the hospital... Well, me being in the room freaked her out, because she was like, 'I can't do one more thing with you, mom.'

"But with Mike, she knew that there was someone there who would respect her, and that calmed her down.

"So, seeing me made her even more anxious. So, I retreated and went away from her into a different room, and Mike and Cat Chow were in the bedroom, and he was able to make her calm.

"And I don't even know what he does, but after a little while, over the course of a day, he was able to calm her down, so that she was then able to be herself again..."

CHAPTER EIGHTEEN

Hot Springs for medicinal purposes...

Before I could share that my relationship with Cat Chow was all derived from teachings I had acquired from Phillip, the call got dropped because of reception difficulties as we reached the snow-covered summit of the Bighorn Mountains pass between Montana and Wyoming.

I asked how Phillip got involved in the hot spring matter in Thermopolis? He said that when he was starting to have his health problems, and he was going to the doctors and wasn't getting better, he went to the Wind River Reservation to pick cedar for medicinal purposes, just as he and his family had done for generations.

Then, they went to the Hot Springs for medicinal purposes, as well, and Nicole read a petition about the hot springs, and talked with a lifeguard, and asked if they'd involve the tribes?

When he said they hadn't, Nicole and Phillip made arrangements to meet with the owner of the hot springs, Roland.

From there, they got things rolling to support the Hot Springs as a place where all tribal people could enjoy and appreciate, just to say they'd done for most of their history...

CHAPTER NINETEEN

Swimming in the Hot Springs...
Tuesday, October 21, 2025

Nicole told me that Phillip had difficulty sleeping during the night, and suggested that we let him sleep late, and go out ourselves and investigate the Hot Springs.

Talking, she validated a number of my concerns, as pertained to continuing Phillip's legacy.

When Phillip woke, he, Nicole and I climbed the Faces Mountain. On the ascent, we looked out at the lovely fall colors coming from the trees in the valley below us. But I noted that Phillip was getting easily winded and had balance difficulties, so that I effectively caught him a couple of times to keep him from falling.

Raising the subject of continuing his legacy, Phillip shared a Kumbaya idea that he was going to arrange an event similar to the Sundance before the little bighorn battle, in which he brought his children together and instructed them to carry on the organization he'd built.

After coming down from the mountain, we went to the hot springs center, where I met the Tribal President of the Wind River Reservation and his wife and grandson, as well as Roland, the owner of "Star Plunge", which was the main hot springs center.

Swimming in the Hot Springs was the highlight of the trip for me. It was an absolute delight to be in that water, which I enjoyed to the fullest.

After swimming, we had dinner at Roland's home. He was an extremely gracious host and treated the tribal elders from the Wind

River Reservation with the utmost humility and care...

CHAPTER TWENTY

False hope?...
Wednesday, October 22, 2025

The following morning in Thermopolis, while Phillip was still sleeping, Nicole invited me to return to Roland's. There, I met Roland's daughter, Taylor, who was nursing her newborn son. I was immediately taken by her, finder her a very warm and caring person and had great hopes that she'd help navigate divides and bridge the gaps between the tribes and white Thermopolis community when it came to the Hot Springs, and make a difference in so many lives!

She was aware of Phillip's cancer, and she told me that she'd had a grandmother who also had metastatic colon cancer.

"She had all kinds of invasive procedures to treat it," she said. "Surgery to remove the cancer from her colon, lobectomy of the liver to remove liver metastasis, radiation to the lungs.

"What ultimately got her was it spread to her brain, and then, it was over; and even with everything they did to her, she only survived for two years."

Nodding, I considered the fact that only treatment Phillip was receiving was chemotherapy, and his five-year survival prognosis was 10%...

CHAPTER TWENTY-ONE

Here for a purpose...

Roland and Taylor invited Nicole and me back to the Hot Springs to swim. Nicole wanted to find the goggles that had gone missing yesterday (which belonged to the grandson of the Tribal President). I typically don't like to spend a lot of time underwater, because breath holding triggers my near drowning experience from my youth in that undertow; but then I decided that this was an opportunity for me to lean into my trauma, and potentially process and reconcile it, so I helped look for the lost googles; and ultimately, the more tightness I felt in my chest, the more I decided I needed to do underwater swimming.

I had confided to Nicole about my friend, Sam, and she made the connection that the two of us shared issues of breathing.

She couldn't have been more right, as Sam had experienced a near drowning experience a thousand-fold worse than my own...

After swimming, we collected Phillip at the hotel and drove into the Wind River Reservation. There, we went to a site near the river to pick cedar that had been a family tradition for generations...

After that, we got on the road back to go back to Montana. As we drove, I told Phillip that I'd reviewed the book that he and Nicole had been working on, as well as the articles in the Guardian that they'd published, and felt that the wider dominant white culture had to be assisted when it came to Phillip's offering about Indian thinking; that is, he was referring to Native American thinking as circular, and I told him that that had a negative connotation, and needed to be described in other ways, like holistic or integrative.

Phillip accepted these recommendations, which Nicole appreciated, because she'd previously raised this issue with Phillip and hadn't been able to convince him...

I tried to discuss Phillip's condition, saying I understood he did not want to discuss his prognosis, however, it was my opinion that as well as hoping for the best, he also had to prepare for the worst, and felt he had to become more like a foreman or a contractor delegating to others the work on his land, because it was too physically taxing for a person with advanced cancer.

"I'll do it for as long as I feel I'm up to it," he insisted.

I tried to share about what happened to Sam, and how his lung condition overtook him all at once. Then, I made the mistake of confiding about my difficulty reconciling what I saw in that last dream about Sam.

"Your thoughts and energy and spirit," he began. "They're connected. And you can create thoughts and you can erase them and replace them. We have that ability.

"So, all these thoughts that are connected to trauma, to the dark side... If you can create them, and you can think them, you can reverse that. And you can erase them, and be kind and merciful, with empathy.

"Those thoughts that you're having are merely old programming, and now it's up to you to learn and unlearn and relearn, and reset and reboot and shift your perception and shift you're thinking and go downwards to upwards in energy."

I told Phillip that where I could agree with him on most things, when it came to erasing thoughts and memories and trauma, then I disagreed, saying I thought it was more important to reconcile trauma than to erase it – because when we reconcile our experiences of trauma, they make us stronger.

But Phillip effectively disagreed, and instead insisted on taking me through an exercise of erasure.

"Close your eyes," Phillip insisted. "Close your eyes. Now, rub your hands, back-and-forth.... Now, rubbing your hands is an imaginary tool to wipe away stuff. OK?

"Now, you can't get to it through your left brain. You can only get to it from pure awareness. Spiritual awareness. In the right brain. Are you with me?... Visualize a Red box. Tell me when you're there. Now erase it. Rub your hands. There you go. Visualize a blue dot. Now erase that. Rub your hands and erase that. OK, now, I need you to visualize an oak tree with big old leaves and a stream of water running beside it, with luscious tall grass, and smells like mint tea. Now, there's trout going back-and-forth, and it's shallow, clearer, blue water. Can you see all of them? Can you smell all of that? And this is happening under a clear full moon night.

"Now, there's a Red box sitting under the trunk of that tree trunk. Now erased all of that. Now, all what you've done is prove to me that you can visualize and erase it and replace it with a new thought.

"So, now, close your eyes, and I want you to take some of your thoughts that are related to 'can't' and 'but' and 'hopelessness', 'pressure', worry', fear', 'abandonment'... Can you see some of those thoughts coming at you? OK, erase all of those thoughts.

"Now, replace them with a happy thought, like what you love the most as a child. What made you really happy as a child. What makes you really happy now. Now erase that. Now, tell me the worst that's happened to you when it's come to people. Tell me when you get there. Now erase that. Now erased that with those happy thoughts about certain people.

"Now, no matter how you happy you can get with those certain people, or those certain thoughts, you'll never reach this place. I'm going to take you to. Because those happy thoughts are connected to your bad thoughts, and your bad thoughts are connected to your good thoughts, and the good people are connected to those bad people.

"But let's go to another place that anytime those bad worries, fears, poor thoughts start to come, you need to erase them. You need to run them away and replace them with good thoughts.

"And then once you come to a good place of a good thought, then I need you to wipe that good thought away, because no matter how good that thought was, it's still connected to that other place.

"Now, when she comes to that good thought place, erase that good thought place..."

All of this was going to the kind of worse connotation in circular thinking that I felt like I was concerned about with his model.

"So, we just got through rebooting you, because you're only capable of thinking so many thoughts in a day, so many thoughts in an hour, so many thoughts in a minute. But the problem is, it's the same thoughts that you thought two or three days ago. even an hour ago. Even five minutes ago.

"So, in order for you to reboot yourself, you have to continue to replace, erase, and replace your thoughts.... And move to this place of no thought, because it will allow you new thoughts to come in."

"Now, what did you get out of that exercise?" he asked.

Your theory, I responded, flippantly.

"Well, it's going to become your new reality," he said, forcefully. "It has to. If we're gonna make a change in this world. We have to meet there where there's no thought.

"Because we need new thoughts. We don't need Einstein theories. We don't need Elon Musk theories, or Donald Trump theories, or Biden theories. We need new thoughts that are going to make upward lasting change.

"And we are the best vessel of that. And if you don't think. That you're capable of changing this world, you are wrong. Somebody damaged your programming, by putting in programming with doubt, fear, shame, and angst."

It wasn't that I doubted that I was capable of those kinds of changes – Indeed, I felt I was working towards it.

"You are," he affirmed. "You're there. You're open to it."

I described the last moments with my friend Sam, and what I felt I got out of that vision – which was the feeling that, in spite of how difficult the end was, and maybe how difficult that person's life was through it, you're going to accept going through that experience again, because you spend enough time in the darkness and you're going to be willing to attempt that kind of suffering if it's you're only option.

"And, therefore, it leads me to think that, even though I am moving towards the spiritual world, and I've had my life, and I don't need to be invested in this physical plane as much anymore, because I'm going somewhere else, and I don't have any kids... Well, there's a reason to be invested in this physical plane," I said, "and that's because the physical plane and the spiritual plane are connected, and therefore there is a reason to always want to make things better."

"I don't believe in reincarnation," Phillip declared. "But I do believe in organons. Do you know what organons are? When you breathe in, let out, you're putting out organon into the world. And we are breathing and inhaling Jesus, Sitting Bull, Hitler, Donald Trump, all the human and animals and spirits that put these organs into the atmosphere, that's trapped in here.

"That's the closest I can come to reincarnation. I really believe that we are spirits having a human experience. And that the last breath that we take here is the first breath that we're going to take on the other side.

"I was told as a child to look towards the Milky Way; and there's going to be white speckles and light and energy coming; and the further that I move up, I'm going to become one with the Creator and my ancestors when I cross over to the other side, because all my relatives are there waiting.

"White people call it, 'The happy hunting grounds.' But there's no heaven or hell. We make our own heaven or hell right here. Because my journey and my future is inside of me. It's not external; it's internal. And I'm not going to let fear and shame and guilt and condemnations get in the way of that – Because I know that they're all man-made.

"So, the inward journey defines the outward journey. That's the new future. Just like the new dyslexia of the 21st century is the ones that learned one way and can't unlearn that way and relearn another way. And when you start to change, then it's inevitable. You cannot hang onto the lower level and expect to go to a higher level.

"And you are right there. Because, believe me, I know… Hell or heaven. Alive or dead. I love you. I really enjoy today with you. I really enjoyed watching you. Pick and prune the cedar. And watching you in the water, swimming like a salmon. And in the leaves changing, and just being in your presence. Because I truly believe that you are here for a …"

CHAPTER TWENTY-TWO

Prayers for Cat Chow...

At the very moment when Phillip was about to complete his sentence, I got a call from April...

CHAPTER TWENTY-THREE

Cat Chow getting worse...

Long story short, Cat Chow passed away...

CHAPTER TWENTY-FOUR

Yellow Horse shirt...

At present, April wants to keep these moments private...

CHAPTER TWENTY-FIVE

Doing worse…

So, for now, I'm removing the contents of these chapters…

CHAPTER TWENTY-SIX

Need to be a part of the moment?

The Cat Chow-inspired dynamic Qi Gong self-practice that came out of our interaction during the mourning process April did want shared...

CHAPTER TWENTY-SEVEN

Memories of Cat Chow as a kitten...

That will start at Chapter Thirty-six...

CHAPTER TWENTY-EIGHT

Arriving at Phillip's home...

...

CHAPTER TWENTY-NINE

"It" was happening...

...

CHAPTER THIRTY

"Paying the price..."

...

CHAPTER THIRTY-ONE

Events have overtaken us...

...

CHAPTER THIRTY-TWO

Cat Chow finds her voice...

...

CHAPTER THIRTY-THREE

Plans for dying moments...

...

CHAPTER THIRTY-FOUR

"Messengers?..."

...

CHAPTER THIRTY-FIVE

"Fighting to the end..."

...

CHAPTER THIRTY-SIX

Dantian & motherhood...

April picked me up at the airport and drove me back to the house.

In the living room, Cat Chow lay peacefully in a coffin on top of her cat tower, which had been with us since she was a kitten.

"It's so hard to think that we will take her away from the house," April commented, tearfully.

As soon as I connected energetically with Cat Chow, it was as though the energy were directing me to the ground on my hands and knees, as though it were now my time to be on all fours?

Meanwhile, April said that she was experiencing a feeling of energy at her Dantian.

The Dantian is the vital energy center about 3 inches below the navel, representing the vestigial umbilical cord, from which we first received nourishment and oxygen within the womb and effectively took breath.

It happened that I had an experience not unlike April when my mother passed away: Standing at my mother's side at the mortuary, I connected with my mother energetically and experienced a feeling energy at my Dantian for the first time.

"This is my mother," the feeling seemed to say.

Now, I asked April if she had ever felt anything like this before?

"No," she said, definitively. "This has never happened to me before."

I commented that perhaps April's feeling of energy at her Dantian made sense because she was like Cat Chow's mom?

"Yeah, Cat Chow, you made me into a mom," she said. "Thank you for allowing me to experience motherhood..."

CHAPTER THIRTY-SEVEN

Sacrifice in exchange for 'The Cat Chow'...

April braided her hair, then asked me to cut it, just as we'd done for Ini.

"I want her to go to the next phase with a part of me," she said.

I cut her hair, and we laid it in its braid next to Cat Chow. It seemed like Cat Chow's fur was melding into April's, and its color lightening, so to leave me wondering whether, in the next life, Cat Chow would come back as a blonde?

"She would say, 'Thank you, mom, for giving me that gift'," April commented. "You could see that it's kind of shining on hers, and where our hair is mingling with the way the light is hitting it – It looks like it's becoming brown."

"Mingling with a mother's love, and a daughter's love," she added. "You know, I'm giving her my youth. Because now the hair that's growing out has a lot more white."

"So, that was a real sacrifice, "she declared. "It was my little Sundance, I guess."

Then, she turned and cried and asked me to perform a ceremony, in which I connect energetically with Cat Chow, as we'd done with Ini; and requesting that we performed it in the bedroom, where she'd last cuddled with Cat Chow.

"I should have just stayed that way longer," she said, "but I didn't know if would be the last time."

So, we positioned the cat tower with Cat Chow's coffin in the bedroom, like an altar, from which I would interact, while April lay in the bed.

Connecting with Cat Chow energetically, April again said she was experiencing a feeling of energy at her Dantian.

"I am also feeling it at the third eye," she said.

And that was exactly where I was feeling energy, as well as around my eyes.

"But the Dantian is stronger," she added.

I was feeling the energy strongly in my hands. So strongly that when my hands move past and crossing my face, I could feel the energy radiating out from them, which was not typical.

Where my hands were concerned, I was feeling energy intensely and very, definitely in my first three fingers, thumb, index finger, but most strongly in the middle finger.

Then, I followed the energy in my hands downwards into a squat, and it struck me how easily and fluidly I was able to go into it. There was no problem of balance at all. It was just effortless.

As I remained in that squatting position, my hands were near my scalp, so that the energies were interacting there.

Again. I couldn't believe how balanced I was.

Then, I stood up from that squat, and it was so easy that I couldn't help from saying, "No sweat."

And to my surprise, my chest felt more opened. And this was really mysterious to me, because when I was in that squat, my chest was compressed against my legs?...

I squatted again, and then stood upright again, no sweat.

I was feeling energy intensely, solidly, at my third eye, right there at the bridge of my nose.

I went down again into a squat, and I was so capable of staying in that position that it was like I'd been doing it all my life, as though I'd grown up in an indigenous or Asian culture where it was commonplace. And these were neither muscles nor positions that Americans were used to assuming. How is it now so easy for me?

Minute seven

Down again into a squat, then rising. And I was becoming aware of a pattern: I would follow the energy in my hands forward, so to advance my shoulders and head, and that momentum took me downwards into the squat; and then that same forward movement would give me the momentum to easily take me upwards into a standing position again.

And, again, my chest was feeling more open.

Minute eight

The energy mostly left my hands, though I did feel a lingering sensation, especially in the line between my middle finger to the base of my thumb, all the way to the tip; the energy still very strong at my third eye at the bridge of my nose.

Then the energy came back to my hands again, move them and my shoulders and head forwards, and took me into that squad again.

Now, my shoulders were supported at the knees by the armpits, and it was holding me very securely in that squat position, with my head between my knees.

Then, with a slight lean forward, I easily stood upwards from the squat again, no sweat.

And again, my chest was feeling very open.

Minute 10

Went into another squat, and this time, my body leaned back slightly, until it was time for me to pull it forward, so I didn't fall backwards, the momentum sending me standing again. This was more physically challenging than anything in the experience thus far.

And standing, the energy had me leaning forwards a bit, which was also more physically challenging then had been other things in this experience.

Now, my hands followed the energy in an arching fashion upwards to the sky, as though making an offer offering to the universe, and then the energy directed my hands to move my arms downwards and out again.

Went into another squat, and this time, my arms were close to my knees, and my hands interacting with the energy at my crown chakra.

Standing upright from the squat, my hands were still connected with the crown chakra, so that as my head moved from a bowed position to an upright position, my hands followed, still connected energetically with the crown chakra.

Next, my hands expanded outwards to both sides, just feeling like I was opening up energetically to everything everywhere, and the energy at my hands and my crown chakra just sharing my energy everywhere, totally connected energetically with the universe.

Next, my hands went straight out from my shoulders, like Jesus on the cross, though my palms were directed upwards.

The energy in my hands directing my arms downwards towards my body, my elbows first contacting my body, then my hands.

My hands moved upwards over my chest and then downwards, and I could feel the energy from my hands radiating out and interacting with my chest, which felt like it was opening up.

Then, my heels clicked together. My feet had already been close to each other throughout this. Now, the angle of the heels was maybe 45°.

I could feel energy now between my hands and first chakra at the genital area.

My body arced downwards at the angle of my back, until my body went into a squat; my arms were straight out with my hands, relatively close to the ground and sending energy into the Earth, mostly coming from those first three fingers, particularly the middle finger, followed by the thumb and index finger.

Leaning forward slightly, the moment stood me upright, effortlessly, my back straightening out last.

The energy was still very strong at my third eye, and I felt very open at my chest and relaxed at my shoulders.

My heels were still together, my feet angled 45°. My knees bent a little bit as it felt like I was sinking into my feet.

Then, I felt directed to put weight on the left foot, which is a problem, in general, as that foot is very tight, and I'm usually not able to put weight on it.

I'd been facing Cat Chow, but my body was turning me now to face the wall.

It was dusk now, and I could appreciate the gold highlights of April's hair against Cat Chow's black fur.

My hands were connecting energetically with my chest, and my hands moved across my torso.

I found that I was standing more erect, so that my head was really upright and my eyes directed straight ahead.

I felt the energy directing me clockwise to face the sliding glass door, as though taking me into the future and following the sun, and not unlike my last experiences with Ini.

Standing, I felt really grounded. With the left foot, I felt this stretch across the medial aspect, which seemed to be trying to heal from all those years of my trying to create that artificial arch to try to please my father, or fit into shoes that were too small and tight for that foot.

I followed an inner intelligence directing minute movements in my feet, up and down, and being directed towards the left foot in a slight counterclockwise direction. Again, there was that feeling of sinking into the left foot, like I was trying to stretch it, especially across the medial arch.

I thought about Cat Chow, who always had the best balance and most graceful walk; and how it was for a 10-pound little cat, when she walked on me, I felt intense pressure with her steps, so to indicate just how grounded she was.

I continued to move in slow and infinitesimal, counterclockwise movements – my right foot rising and stepping, but my left foot was mostly pivoting. I was going around and around and around in very slow revolutions. My eyes closed, I wondered in which direction I would end up facing?

I could really feel that stretch in my left foot.

Minute 25

My hands up to above my head, feeling energy in my hands, especially in the middle index and thumb fingers, my hands descended, following a line of the energy like a beam or pole coming up from my crown chakra, then down to my head and ears.

My fingers were all spread out, and I was still pivoting around my left foot counterclockwise.

I was feeling very grounded, especially in my hips. I had most of my weight off of my right foot, and I was standing in something of a ballet plié position, like a ballerina, most of the weight on my left foot.

Finally, it felt like a lot of the energy was discharging from my hands and head, and opening my eyes, I found that all of those counterclockwise turns had stopped with my facing April.

April had fallen into a sleep.

I was still feeling some residual energy at my upper third eye.

The energy led me to raise my hands, so that the palms were facing April and in proximity to either side of my mouth.

My arms were directed downwards, till my elbows were at my sides, followed by my hands at my sides.

Then, my arms went up again with my palms directed towards April, as though sending energy her way.

Next, my hands were directed downwards until I could feel they were energetically connected with my first chakra/genital area, and then extending outward towards April, and then, I bent low, as though to bowing towards April. Then, I squatted all the way down. Then, with a lean forward of my head and shoulders, I rose till I was finally upright.

I could feel some residual energy in my fingers, especially the middle finger, then index finger and thumb. There was energy at my third eye. I was still facing April. Most all of my weight was on my left foot, as those stretching that arch area.

I bent my knees, mostly my left knee, where I was putting my weight, and then went into another squat, in which most the weight was on that left foot, so that I'd say it was 75% left foot, 25% right.

With a slight forward movement, I was directed upwards from the squat, with the back last to straighten.

I felt like my chest was really open, which really surprised me, because each time I went to a squad, it felt like I was collapsing my chest. Was collapsing a form of stretching?

Again, I was taken in a counterclockwise direction, pivoting with the left foot, and stepping with the right, moving very slowly.

I was directed to arch my back backwards, so that my hips were thrust somewhat forward.

Then, to my surprise, I was directed to pivot in the clockwise direction, still feeling the stretch in the sole of the left foot, where all the weight was, while the right foot felt really light, like the body wasn't putting any weight on it.

And it struck me that this was really different for me, because when I walk, it feels like I'm only putting weight on my right foot, and my left foot is never grounded, so I'm just falling on it while it's in an inverted position.

My pelvis arced so that I was putting my butt out, which was not at all natural for me. I was still putting most of my weight on my left foot, keeping my right foot very light on the ground.

Next, my hips were directed to sway this way in that. Sway to the right, sway to the left. Over and over, still feeling the stretch mostly in my left foot.

It felt like this practice was especially meant for me to help stretch out that left foot.

And I was really feeling my sacrum moving in a way that I don't think I'd ever felt before: I was still feeling more movement on the right side, whereas the left felt locked, but moving incrementally, like things were on their way to opening up there.

I continue to sway my hips left and right.

April was really sleeping now, snoring.

My chest felt really open, and I was standing straight.

My hands are upwards over my head, so that I was standing with energy leaving my hands, especially active at the tip of my middle finger, index finger and thumb.

I could feel energy at my upper third eye and a bit at my crown chakra.

I sank into my body with my knees bent, feet mostly together, feeling very grounded and balanced, and a general feeling of relaxation everywhere in my body - especially noticeable was the feeling of relaxation in my chest, which I typically do not experience. I just felt good.

My hands forward, I went again in a bow, this time with my knees slightly bent, and then arched all the way down into a squat, so that my head was mostly at my knees.

I was directed upwards again, starting at the lower back as a fulcrum and then moving upwards, one vertebrae at a time.

The energy left my hands, but was still there at my third eye and crown chakra.

I bent low into another bow, mostly with my lower back is a fulcrum and bending my knee slightly and into a squat, until my head was close to my knees again. And then I was directed upwards again like before.

Minute 37

The weight was still mostly on my left foot, as I sank mostly into my left foot.

My third eye was very active. It was literally like a connection between my third eye and left foot, like I was left to think, "I had to artificially arch my feet, because my father said it was a matter of survival. He said that if you had flat feet, your tire easier. So, I needed arches." And I was integrating that trauma at my third eye, which was the chakra that reconciled our higher ideals with our need for survival.

Hence, higher ideals would tell me to just love my body, like, "Everything is OK. Everything is good in the world", as opposed to my father, who was sending a message saying, "No, everything is all wrong with you."

Opening my chest way out, arching my back forward, feeling the stretch in my left foot, though now the weight is more evenly distributed between the two feet.

Arching forward slightly, going down into another squat, with most of the weight on that left foot, I was being slightly supported by the bed, which was to the right of me.

Now, I was directed forward and then rising to a stance.

Minute 39

The energy was mostly out of my hands, my hands being directed towards the sky in an arcing fashion.

There was lots of energy at my third eye.

My hands are now being directed downwards, my chest really open.

It seemed counterintuitive that all of the squatting was relaxing my chest so much?

Then, a "pop" occurred at my left ankle, like an adjustment there, so that I felt like I was standing, able to bear weight at the medial aspect of that ankle, so to feel more secure and grounded in the left ankle than I think ever before. There's still a stretch across the arch of my left foot, from the heel to the first metatarsal. It just felt like I was really grounded in that left foot, and this was a first in the way of my ever standing like this.

The energy directing me into another squat, most of the energy on my left foot.

Now the energy was directing me back, until instead of rising from the squat, I was directed to sit on the floor.

I could feel energy leaving my hands and going into the ground, like I was letting a lot of Turbid chi go into the ground, and I could feel relaxed, sitting there happily on the ground, supporting myself slightly against the bed on my right side.

I could feel a slight stretch involving my medial left handspring and medial aspect of my left leg.

Minute 43

The energy was directing me to lay back against the ground.

I was feeling a lot of stretching, especially along the left side of me, especially at my sacrum. It just felt way open, very easy to expand.

My neck still felt tight, like it was in this curved semicircle created by the cervical spines. (Of note, connecting with Cat Chow energetically would ultimately relieve this difficulty at my neck on the following day, when the universal Chi would take volitional control and stretch my neck to the left side and then to the right, first with my head level, then with my neck upwards and bent 45°, then with my head bent more so that I was turning with my face upwards one side and then the other.)

My left hip still felt rather achy, and the energy directed them side to side while still lying on the ground. Left sacrum belt rather tight, but loosening.

I felt some tight aspects of my buttocks on the left, connected with the left sacrum.

Now, I was directed to relax and stop moving. I felt muscular releases on the medial aspect of my left foot between the heel and ankle.

Then, I let out a spontaneous exhalation that seemed to signal the end of this Qi Gong exercise that Cat Chow's energy had inspired, so that I felt the need to get up now.

And I felt really even, with just the slightest tension in the media aspect of the sole of my left foot, but, otherwise, balanced and grounded.

Lifting my feet from side to side, I felt like I was enjoying a new experience, with less tension in the shoulders and back, with my head held high.

There was some residual feeling of energy in my fingers, as well as my third eye.

I was now feeling intense energy at my crown chakra, which just felt like a definite feeling of energy there - a tingling at the top of my head, which I hadn't felt in a while, as, of late, I'd been feeling the energy in my head much more in my upper third eye than my crown chakra.

But now I was feeling that tingling at my crown chakra. It was unmistakable. I don't think I've felt this since the beginning of the long Covid-Qi Gong project with that first group. And at that time, with that first group, it seemed like I was feeling that crown chakra because I needed the universal Qi to help me with these patients who were suffering from a condition that I had no experience, so that I needed the universal blueprint.

And maybe where all of this was concerned with all of this new integration and helping me come to terms with the trauma that my father inspired, I needed the universal chi for that, too?

It just felt like this whole cat chow-energy inspired exercise opened up that tight band of muscle along the arch of left foot, so that I could stand on that foot.

Minute 50

I was feeling energy across my chest, especially the pectoralis muscles, and into the center of my chest, at my heart, so that it felt more open.

It just felt like I was walking around like people do when they feel good, like they don't have a care in the world, head up, feeling happy and gay. Shoulders way back, everything just felt like it was kind of working.

And I was sinking into my left foot like never before and just felt like if I did this every day, I would just get better and better, and be way better off. Cat Chow had given me the way.

"Cat Chow sure knew how to be healthy in her stance and posture," April said, "so that her body flowed so correctly. She did the cat walk really well."

Yes, and it felt like she had just imparted a lot of that to me. She had given me an exercise so that with time and practice, I could do the cat walk just as well.

I asked April to take a photo of me in my new Cat Chow-inspired posture.

Looking at the photo, it felt like I was standing straight up and down, with my head squarely on top of my neck, and not forward leaning at all.

And that is the Cat Chow Qi Gong practice, and I think if I do it every day, like I said, I'll be in a lot better shape...

CHAPTER THIRTY-EIGHT

"Focused on giving..."

April shared about her mindset during the practice.
"I was focused on giving," she said. "On being loving. That's what I wanted to do. I wanted to give her that."
April talked about how it was that she had put herself in the position when Cat Chow last cuddled with her.
"I should have just stayed that way," she said, regretting her previous actions.
Then, she directed her comments to Cat Chow, "I didn't know, Cat Chow, that it would be the last time. But I felt like I tried to give it to you again right now."
"I regret the sleeping," she added, "but that happens to me with Qi Gong."
I said it was my experience that rest is so important to healing, so I wasn't bothered by that.
"And she loved to sleep," she commented. "She spent a lot of time sleeping."
Meanwhile, April reported that she was already experiencing less heartburn, and I wondered that Cat Chow imparted some healing to her that way and hoped it would continue, and maybe this physical practice would help April, too...

CHAPTER THIRTY-NINE

"...if you want to be graceful..."

April got up and felt inspired to attempt to squat like I had and asked me to squat with her. I stood with my feet slightly apart, heels essentially together, and then felt the energy at my hands become active, which directed me slightly forward at my shoulders and head, so that I then bent slightly forward at my back and went from there easily into a squatting position.

Then, coming out of that, I just followed the energy at my hands as it again took me forward slightly, with my shoulders and head following and putting momentum into my body, I followed that upwards from the squat to a standing position, with a final arching at my back to stand upright.

"You're impressive," April said. "You can do it with your feet flat on the ground. I don't have that flexibility at my ankles."

It was hard to imagine myself an impressive physical specimen, as it seemed a contradiction, as for my whole life I was considered, as my father would say, "gimpy."

But April persisted and made the comment that since the Cat Chow-inspired practice, I'd immediately been moving more gracefully.

"So, this is 'The Cat Chow'," she declared. "This is 'The Cat Chow practice.' We can do The Cat Chow every morning. We can do it together.

"She's like, 'Hey, if you want to be graceful like me, do The Cat Chow'..."

CHAPTER FORTY

Different variations...

"Do you want to repeat the practice?" April asked.

Probably a good idea, I said. Let's do it.

Cat Chow was still present in the room on her cat tower, but rather than connect with her energetically, I simply connected with the energy at my hands, which directed them forward, until my head and shoulders followed, until my body was directed downwards into a squat.

Squatting, the energy in my hands was flowing to the ground; until what time I was pulled back, then forwards, which imparted just the right amount of momentum to help me effortlessly rise to a standing position, up with my legs and then up with my back, till I'm standing upright.

And then I found that the energy in my hands were directing them to the sky, and I felt this opening at my crown chakra, so that both of my hands could feel the beam of energy coming from the Crown chakra; then, I effectively slid my hands down that beam, and followed the energy down the sides of my head, until I opened my hands outwards, my elbows at my sides, till my hands came to rest at my slides.

And this all happening without my connecting with Cat Chow energetically at all - She had just catalyzed this practice. Now, I was able to do it on my own. My system was open to this practice. Like I'd received a download and could now do it on my own.

minute eight

With another squat, after sending energy into the ground, my hands were directed upward to interact with my crown chakra, before the energy directed me forward, and the momentum led me to stand again.

In this way, I was recognizing different variations of this dynamic internal Qi Gong self-practice, with some generalizations I felt I could recognize:

Number one, both to enter the squat and to rise from it, follow the energy as it slightly tilts the body forward, to give the momentum needed to enter those positions, either downwards for the squat or upwards to stand.

Second, after raising them to follow the energy from the crown chakra, first bring the elbows to the side, then the hands to the side...

CHAPTER FORTY-ONE

Cat Chow ways...

After the Cat Chow practice, April suggested we take a walk. As we walked, I found that my ambulating was improved, with a willingness to pronate when toeing off with my left foot off using my first metatarsal, instead of supinating into the ankle, which had been my general, dysfunctional pattern. Now, I was now walking with my feet firmly planted on the ground. It all left me feeling like a lot of love and healing was imparted to me through the self-practice that Cat Chow inspired.

April was disappointed about Phillip's attitude towards Cat Chow.

"He's succumbed to the sickness that he was trying to fight," she said. "Sell his horses. 'Don't have any feeling for cats... They don't matter... The only thing that matters are human beings.'"

She shook her head.

"I think it might be because he's in survival mode and things kind of got hard for him," she offered. "It sounds like he's lost a lot... It sounds like his kids aren't taking over, and he has more and more work, so I can understand why he wants to sell the horses.

"So, it might be that his horses are better off, as long as he can find good buyers and he's not selling them to get slaughtered."

Phillip had expressed that concern, especially with his best horses.

"How many horses does Phillip have?" April asked.

Maybe 20, I said.

"I guess they're not all Sioux Boy," she commented, referring to the horse with whom he we train children in native horsemanship.

"So, these four horses were just a small percentage of what he has left. Who is helping him keep up everything?"

The high school student, Mike, was helping, but, in general, it seemed like it was mostly on him.

His son, Smiley, was a big help with the four horses on Thursday morning, as well as taking me to the airport.

I thought Smiley was a really sturdy fella, who would probably be the best of Phillip's family members I met to take over. Nicole had said something to this effect, as well.

When he took me to the airport, he thoughtfully asked about Cat Chow...

CHAPTER FORTY-TWO

"Love is shining..."

Returning to the house, April admired the braid against Cat Chow's fur.

"It's like shining on her," she said. "My hair is shining. Shining on her. Love is shining..."

Then, she turned and cried and held me...

CHAPTER FORTY-THREE

"Baksheesh…"

Just then, April's sister, Yael, sent a text, saying, "May she be at peace while somehow also free to frolic on adventures."

She added, "I was honored to have that time with her, seeing her strong and bright spirit."

"Not bad for a little kitten who we took in, injured, and malnourished because she was internally infected with worms, who was brave enough to walk through that door and trust and take that leap of faith," April said. "That was Cat Chow. She was just so strong. Her will."

I reminded her that, at the time, it did take an offering of some milk to convince Cat Chow to go through that threshold and, hence, required some coaxing.

"She needed a little baksheesh," April responded. "Especially now that we know Cat Chow. She's no dummy…"

CHAPTER FORTY-FOUR

"Jewish automatically..."

Completing our ceremonies, we smudged and sang prayers and psalms, then prepared to take Cat Chow to the referral center until burial arrangements were made.

"Even in her death pose, she's such an elegant girl," April commented of her. "She is totally a cat walker. Even in death, she aces the cat walk."

Taking a photo, April castigated me, saying that it was forbidden in Jewish law.

When I responded that Cat Chow wasn't Jewish, April begged to differ.

"She was Jewish," she insisted. "Her mother was Jewish and that made her Jewish automatically..."

CHAPTER FORTY-FIVE

"OK to let go..."

Arriving at the Referral Center, before entrusting Cat Chow to the staff, I interacted with her energetically not once but twice – and on both occasions had an energetic experience that essentially said, "It's OK to let go."

Indeed, in the second one, it seemed to be saying that, although Cat Chow's work was done, I still had work to do – and doing that work was what was important. That's why I'm still here.

As for Cat Chow, I think she achieved what she was put here to do; and she would say, "Thanks, mom and dad, I had a great life. I thoroughly enjoyed it. I well exceeded any expectations for a cat and what a cat is supposed to be capable of. I loved every moment with you guys. You were extremely good to me. You essentially always honored my wishes..."

CHAPTER FORTY-SIX

"Upgraded..."

Leaving the referral center, April commented about how it was that I hadn't had the best relationship with Cat Chow through most of our time together.

"You weren't bonded," she said of the two of us. "You had to work at a bond."

"For years you had this conflict with her," she continued. "She would pee in inappropriate places and that would cause problems."

Yes, and over the last years, we came a long way, in terms of the little journey that the two of us made together.

"And for the last couple of years, she hasn't done that. It's like she has been really good, and that she put in the effort in her last moments, and then had to pay for it with minutes of gasping for breath... It was like we had this agreement, 'You can stay inside if you pee in the litter box." And she was like, 'I'm going to keep that promise.'"

Yes, in the end, it was much more than keeping a promise – She'd literally give me a path to health!

"In the past two years, she immediately became Ini-like," April commented.

Yes, she certainly was when I was sick with Covid. It was like, "Why is this cat clawing her way into my door and then staying with me all day? Where did this come from? Unconditional love from my cat?"

I wasn't expecting that at all.

"That was an 'Ini move'," I thought.

And I think it heralded the repair of our relationship, so that I made amends, and she made amends, and we had a loving relationship for the past years.

And I really did love her, as evidenced by how much I hurt over losing the house at Mira del Rio because she enjoyed it so much.

And here, at the very end, it seemed she had not only sent me energy of healing, but also energetically guided me through a Qi Gong exercise that I know if I did every day, would just get me better and better.

It was like the saying, "Give a man a fish, and you feed him for a day; teach him how to fish, and you feed him for a lifetime."

That amounted to what connecting with Cat Chow energetically had done.

And all this to say nothing of that last experience, where connecting with her energetically had led to a loss of volitional control to help me facilitate healing at my neck.

"She possibly upgraded you, man," April commented. "We'll see?..."

CHAPTER FORTY-SEVEN

Bobcat encounter...

We decided to honor Cat Chow by taking a walk through our old neighborhood.

First, we walked the block long path by the Mira Del Rio house that we used to take with Ini and Cat Chow in the evenings. Then, April suggested we take a walk along the river and invite Cat Chow's spirit to see a place that she'd never seen before, given that the coyotes there were such that she couldn't ever join us in our walks there with Ini.

I commented again about my last energetic interaction with Cat Chow, when we were trying to decide if we should leave her at the referral center or not? At that time, cat chow's spirit seemed to be telling me that it was OK to let go, and I felt an ease in the discomfort I was feeling at my heart.

"She didn't need to be babied or mothered anymore," April interpreted.

Then, as we were walking, a bobcat appeared on the trail and walked ahead of us.

"And it's walking slow and letting us sort of follow it," April said. "And it's so comfortable with us. It's like not scared at all. And it's like doing what Cat Chow does. Like it's saying, 'See me? I'm going this way. Come follow me', and then it kind of waited a little bit, like he was definitely having us follow him? And he looks so secure. Like so confident. And not aggressive-like... Just self-confident. Like he feels really comfortable on the trail with us here."

We followed the bobcat as it moved along the trail.

"If we were with Ini, I would have turned around and gone home," April said. "It isn't a big bobcat. It's about twice the size of cat chow. We should bring our tobacco and sage and do a little ceremony."

April asked me to sing a Lakota prayer song with her.

"But quietly," she said. "Because we don't want to scare him off or want him to go."

After we were done singing, April said, "Thank you, Cat Chow. Are you in your new form right now? If you are, you certainly don't seem scared right now? A few days ago, if you were walking this path with us, you certainly would be scared. Now, in your new form, your self-confident..."

Being that April was such an excellent scout and so good at following clues and seeing details and knowing which direction to go, we wound up following the bobcat along the trail for a good distance.

Finally, it began to rain, so we had to turn around and make a run for it.

April commented that she thought it was because the bobcat communicated with Cat Chow's spirit, saying, "Friend, I did what you wanted - I sent your message to your people – But those humans of yours are following me, and they're stuck to me like glue, and they won't leave now, and they're making me a little nervous. What are we gonna do about it?"

"So, Cat Chow goes, 'Oh, thank you very much for doing that for me. I'm so sorry they're irritating you now. I think if we make it rain, they'll just go away.' 'So, the bobcat went, 'Oh, then let's just make it rain.'"

And it did rain, and we did go away.

"The story should start, 'Bobcat, help me send a message to my people.' 'Sure, Cat Chow, happy to do it'," April declared. "We always knew that Cat Chow could talk to the dead – Now, maybe she can talk to the living?..."

CHAPTER FORTY-EIGHT

"... even knew a bobcat..."

All the way back to the car, April talked about how it felt like Cat Chow had sent the bobcat as a messenger to say hello.

"Because it was doing the kinds of things that Cat Chow does," April said. "Which would be to turn her head and tell us to follow her. And it was so comfortable in the beginning."

"I've never seen a bobcat in real life like that," April commented, as we ran back to the car. "Have you?"

No, me neither, I said. Not in the twelve years that we'd lived in this neighborhood and walked the river nearly every day, nor any other time.

April laughed.

"We had been saying that we were going someplace where Cat Chow had never been before," she said, "and was getting to learn about it for the first time by following us and sharing with Cat Chow places we went with Ini, while she had to stay confined around the house, and it was like Cat Chow was responding, 'This isn't a strange place for me. I knew it. I even knew a bobcat'..."

CHAPTER FORTY-NINE

Looking towards the Milky Way...

At a campground, I was looking out at the nature and feeling that I was somehow connected with a parallel universe that represented the next life, and Cat Chow and Ini were there...

Awakening from the dream, I recalled my discussions with Phillip regarding the Cheyenne view of the next life.

"I was told as a child to look towards the Milky Way; and there's going to be white specks of light and energy coming; and the further that I move up, I'm going to become one with the Creator and my ancestors when I cross over to the other side, because all my relatives are there waiting..."

April was in the other room and thinking about her, I was filled with feelings of compassion, appreciating who she was, her love of nature, her innocence.

I considered her dyslexia, and how she was teased and harassed as a child. Then, I thought about Phillip, and his learning disabilities and "dyslexia" and issue of being "right-brained", and wondered that that was something April shared with native peoples?

Then, I considered my own difficulties, and how I was pushed to be left-brained, and wondered that that led me to keep my "back up", and have a tendency for being harsh and judgmental; and if I might treat people with compassion and appreciate them for their innocence, like was probably the way of my true nature; and then perhaps I'd perhaps let go of all the neural input holding me locked up in spasms everywhere? Because I have an element of dyslexia, manifested in spelling difficulties, so that when people spell words, I get nervous, so to block my ability to follow.

And as I was thinking all of these things, I experienced spontaneous muscular releases in the left side of my back, which was the main source of trigger points that keep me hung up and unable to be grounded...

Getting up, I went to the living room, where April was on the couch, looking at her computer.

"I've been following Facebook groups that like to go traveling and take photos in California," she said, "and they've been getting beautiful photographs of fall foliage from Yosemite, and I wanted to go, but I didn't want to leave Cat Chow."

Would you like to go now? I asked.

"I feel kind of depressed," she responded, "and I don't think I can get myself to actually get in the car and drive."

I'll drive, I said...

CHAPTER FIFTY

"Signs and symbols..."

We arrived at the Yosemite National Park in time for the sunset, then woke up early for a sunrise walk. Then, as we were crossing a bridge, April spotted another bobcat on the other side of the Merced River.

"Mike, look, it stopped," she said. "And it looking back and then at us, as though frightened. It's obvious that it doesn't want to go back. It wants to go forward. But we're in its way, and it's too nervous about us to continue forward. Let's step back from the railing and let it cross."

We stepped back, and the bobcat jumped on the railing of the bridge and proceeded across and passed right by us. Then, arriving at the other end of the bridge, it looked back at us.

"It's like it wants us to follow it," April said. "How does this happen? That not even a week after Cat Chow's passing that we have these close encounters with bobcats, where we've never, ever, ever seen one in real life before? Could it be that Cat Chow is communicating with these bobcats and getting us to come along?"

We followed it into an old campsite and again, like the last bobcat along the river, April had an uncanny ability of knowing exactly where it was going.

"Oh my God, there it is," she said. "And he looked back, like he was saying, 'Follow me.'"

April turned to me.

"That bobcat was really scared," she said. "But it came to us, and we helped him. He got scared and got on the bridge, but then he didn't want to go through us, and then you moved, and then he was

95

able to go over the railing. That's why I told you to move – So he could exit. Otherwise, he was feeling trapped. It was like it ran right towards us and asked us for help."

Suddenly, tears came to her eyes.

"Cat Chow, you're amazing," she exclaimed. "Thank you, Cat Chow. I miss you, honey. I miss you, too..."

Not long after, we found ourselves in a clearing overlooking the Yosemite Falls.

"Mike, look over there," April said. "It kind of looks like there's a rainbow coming from the falls. Can you see it?"

Absolutely, I could! The rainbow was so large and the colors so intense that it looked like a tremendous Pride flag flowing from the mountain falls.

"Mike, there's a waterfall in Yosemite that's famous for rainbows, and it's really well known, and people will come and look, but this isn't it," April commented. "It's on the other side of the park. And it happens when the sun sets, not at sunrise."

It was definitely there, I responded. Indeed, it was so huge that if I hadn't seen it, I wouldn't have believed it was real and would have thought it was a hoax.

We took some photographs, and then kept moving along the path. But a few steps later, when we looked up again, the falls didn't have the rainbow anymore, and even when we went back to the same place where we'd been standing, it was gone.

"So, that rainbow was in a specific spot at a specific time that was very limited," April exclaimed. "Right after we saw the bobcat. It was just a few minutes after we saw the bobcat."

She shook her head.

"We're getting signs and symbols here," she declared.

Then, she stood back and quoted from the Bible – with her own little twist at the end.

"'People of Israel,'" she said, "'follow me, and I'll show you signs and symbols', from bobcats to rainbows."

Then, she turned to me and smiled.

"I'll tell you, Mike," she said, "it's our girls talking to us. Ini, too..."

ABOUT THE AUTHOR

Michael Yanuck MD PhD is a physician-scientist
whose groundbreaking research at the National Institutes of
Health was the basis for an FDA-approved vaccine for cancer.
Following a traumatic leg injury he returned to medicine. Intent on
caring for the less fortunate, he enlisted in the National Health
Service Corps, worked in urban and rural health centers throughout
the country, then served native peoples in the Indian Health Service.
After three years in the field, he was selected Deputy Director of the
Office of Clinical & Preventive Services at IHS Headquarters.
In 2023 Dr. Yanuck was the recipient of the coveted Science
of Tai Chi & Qigong Award from Harvard University for his
work using BioEnerQi to assist Veterans with problems of
severe traumatic brain injury & neurologic deficits,
chronic pain & opioid dependence, as well as long COVID.
Now, with 30 years' experience in Energy Medicine,
he leads VA efforts to combat the opioid crisis
and advance integrative therapies.